PTCB EXAM
SIMPLIFIED

PHARMACY TECHNICIAN CERTIFICATION EXAM
STUDY GUIDE

BY
DAVID A HECKMAN, PHARMD

PTCB Exam Simplified: Pharmacy Technician Certification Exam Study Guide

ISBN-13: 978-0615883700
ISBN-10: 0615883702

The Pharmacy Technician Certification Board does not endorse or promote this or any other PTCB exam study guide.

The author does not assume and hereby disclaims any liability to any party for losses, damages, and/or failures resulting from an error or omission, regardless of cause.

This publication is not a substitute for legal advice. For legal advice, consult a legal professional.

This publication does not contain actual exam questions.

Book cover created by **Keeling Design & Media, Inc.**

Published by Heckman Media

Printed in the United States of America

To contact the author, e-mail customerservice@pharmacylawsimplified.com

A study guide for the *updated* Pharmacy Technician Certification Exam
The Pharmacy Technician Certification Board announced that the PTCB exam is being reorganized into the following 9 knowledge areas as of November 1st, 2013:

1. Pharmacology for Technicians (13.75%)
2. Pharmacy Law and Regulations (12.5%)
3. Sterile and Non-sterile Compounding (8.75%)
4. Medication Safety (12.5%)
5. Pharmacy Quality Assurance (7.5%)
6. Medication Order Entry and Fill Process (17.5%)
7. Pharmacy Inventory Management (8.75%)
8. Pharmacy Billing and Reimbursement (8.75%)
9. Pharmacy Information Systems Usage and Application (10%)

This study guide contains the information vital to gaining an understanding of each of these knowledge areas in a format that allows you to test yourself as you study. Good luck!

TABLE OF CONTENTS

- $129 exam registration fee.
- Administered at Pearson Vue testing centers.
- Computer-based exam.
- 90 multiple choice questions.
- Basic calculator provided.
- No penalties for guessing.
- 120 minutes to complete.
    - 5 minute introductory tutorial.
    - 110 minute examination.
    - 5 minute exit survey.
- Score range: ~~300 – 900~~. *1,000 – 1,600*
    - Must achieve a score of ~~650~~ or higher to pass. *1400*
        - Answer ~ 70% of questions correct to score 650.

What is an insurance premium?
An insurance premium is the cost of maintaining active insurance coverage (usually charged on a monthly basis). For instance, a company may charge $90/month to provide coverage with a particular plan.

What is a deductable?
A deductable is the amount of money a patient must pay out-of-pocket (in addition to the premium) before the insurance benefits take effect. For instance, let's say Plan A offers 80% co-insurance after a $3,000 annual deductable for a premium of $200/month. In this case, the patient has to record $3,000 worth of out-of-pocket medical expenses (not including the mandatory $200 month premium) before the 80% co-insurance takes effect. In other words, the patient pays 100% of the cost of medical expenses until costs reach $3,000. After costs reach $3,000, then isurance pays 80% of the medical expenses. This cycle repeats annually.

> Note: Typically insurance plans with a higher deductable have a lower premium and vice versa. For example, an insurance company might offer one plan with a $3,000 annual deductable at a premium of $200/month and another plan with a $1,500 annual deductable at $300/month.

What is a formulary?
A formulary is a list of drugs covered under an insurance plan. With many formularies, covered drugs are categorized into tiers. For instance, a cheaper and more effective drug may be listed in tier one and be associated with a lower co-pay than a more expensive and less effective drug listed in tier two or three.

What is a co-payment?
A co-payment (or "co-pay") is an amount of money paid by the insured entity/person in accordane with the terms of the insurance policy. For instance, a prescription drug insurance plan might require the patient to pay a $45 co-pay for brand name prescription drugs and a $10 co-pay for generic prescription drugs. For some plans, instead of charging a fixed dollar amount, the co-payment might be a percentage of the total cost (e.g. a 20% co-payment). A co-payment is an expense that must be assumed by the patient in addition to the insurance premium.

What is an HMO?
An HMO (Health Maintenance Organization) is a type of managed care insurance plan. Managed care plans work by forming agreements with healthcare providers. In the agreement, providers agree to treatment guidelines and reimbursement rates set by the HMO.

How do healthcare providers benefit from an agreement with an HMO?
When a provider's services are covered by an HMO insurance plan, the patients that have those plans are a lot more interested in the provider's service. So, when the provider contracts with an HMO, the demand for the provider's service increases. The provider generates more income from seeing more patients.

What is a PPO?

A PPO (Preferred Provider Organization) is another type of managed care insurance plan. Like an HMO, a PPO will cover medical expenses incurred from healthcare providers and hospitals that have entered into a contract with the PPO. As with an HMO, the provider agrees to certain treatment guidelines and reimbursement rates, and in return the patients with the PPO become interested in the provider's medical services since they are covered by their insurance.

What is CMS?

CMS (Centers for Medicare & Medicaid Services) is the division of the United States Department of Health & Human Services (DHHS) that is responsible for the administration of government health insurance programs such as Medicare, Medicaid, and SCHIP (State Children's Health Insurance Program).

What is a prior authorization?

When an insurance company requires a prior authorization, they are essentially refusing to cover the medication until the rescriber justifies his/her choice of medication. The insurance company wants to verify that it is the right drug for the patient's specific situation. The most common situation where we see prior authorization required is when the prescribed drug is expensive and cheaper alternatives exist. When an insurance company requires prior authorization, the pharmacy notifies the prescriber that a prior authorization is required and he/she must contact the inurance company. Whether or not the prior authorization is completed is not up to the pharmacy, the situation rests between the prescriber and the insurance company. Even after the prescriber has contacted the insurance company, they could still refuse to cover the medication.

What are some reasons an insurance claim might get rejected?
Rejections may occur for a variety of reasons. Listed below are some scenarios in which an insurance company might reject a claim:

- NDC not covered
    - When you try to bill an insurance plan for medications that are not on the formulary, you will get this type of rejection. Typically over-the-counter (OTC) drugs are rejected for this reason.
- Refill too soon
- Therapeutic duplication
- Drug-drug interaction
- Drug utilization review (DUR)
    - Can be overridden if the pharmacist verifies the appropriateness of the prescription.
- Look-alike/sound-alike
    - Some insurance companies will initially reject claims for medications that have error-prone names (like hydralazine and hydroxyzine). This forces the pharmacist to take a closer look at the medication name, reducing the chance of a dispensing error.
- Dose too high
    - When you bill for a days' supply that is too short based on the amount of medication being dispensed and common prescribing practices, the insurance company may reject the claim until you verify the dose with the prescriber and make documentation of the discussion.

Note: when you contact a prescriber's office to clarify any part of a prescription, always document the following information on the prescription hard copy:
1. The detail(s) that was/were verified or changed.
2. The name of the person you spoke with.
3. Time and date of the conversation.
4. Your name or initials.

What is a plan limitation?
Some insurance plans place a plan limitation on certain medications. For instance, a plan may only cover a maximum of 15 tablets of zolpidem in a 30-day time period. With these plans, if you try to bill 16 tablets or more for a 30-days' supply, the claim will be rejected.

What is a PBM?
A PBM (Pharmacy Benefits Manager) is the administrator of the prescription drug portion of many health insurance plans. They are responsible for entering into contracts with pharmacies (a pharmacy must be contracted with a patient's insurance company in order for the patient to use their insurance benefits at that particular pharmacy), developing formularies, and processing prescription drug claims.

What is a Medication Assistance Program (MAP)?
A MAP (Medication Assistance Program) is a program that provides financial help for certain patients that cannot afford their medications.

How do prescription drug coupons work?
Prescription drug coupons must be billed just like insurance plans. Many patients present their drug coupons after the prescription has been filled. This disrupts workflow since you have to process the third party claim again (it is called third party because the customer is one party, the pharmacy is another party, and the insurance or coupon is a third party). If at all possible, always try to get any coupons from the patient when the prescription is first dropped off.

> Note: prescription drug coupons are invalid for patients enrolled in government insurance programs, such as Medicaid or Medicare Part D. Each coupon has fine print (terms & conditions) which may limit a patient's ability to use the coupon (e.g. the fine print might say something like: "patient must be at least 18 years of age").

What is "coordination of benefits?"
Coordination of benefits is a term used for billing more than one third party payer. If someone is covered by two (or more) third party plans, it is important not to bill both plans for the full amount. This would result in overpayment and would be considered insurance fraud. Coordination of benefits ensures that all third parties are billed for the appropriate amount.

What is home health care?
Home health care is basically just what it sounds like, delivery of health care directly in the patient's home. Usually this involves a nurse visiting the patient's home periodically for monitoring and administration of medications (including IV infusions if necessary). An example might be a patient with a bacterial infection of the bone (osteomyelitis) requiring several weeks of IV antibiotic therapy. The patient is initially diagnosed and treated in the hospital, but once stabilized the patient is sent home to receive home health care (for periodic monitoring and infusion of IV antibiotics) for the remaining few weeks of therapy. By receiving therapy at home rather than in the hospital, thousands of dollars in medical expenses are avoided and the outcome for the patient is virtually the same.

What is a home infusion pharmacy?
A home infusion pharmacy is a pharmacy that prepares and delivers medications for administration in the patient's home. These pharmacies typically prepare things like PCA (patient controlled analgesia) pumps, IV antibiotics, IV electrolytes, IM vitamin B12, heparin flushes, TPNs/TNAs, and any other sterile parenteral formulations that might be administered in a patient's home.

> Note: parenteral means introducing something into the body by a route other than the mouth. To break it down, look at the Greek root words: "para-" means aside or beyond, and "-enteral" means pertaining to the intestinal tract.

Dispense as written (DAW) codes make up one piece of information that gets submitted as part of a third party claim (i.e. the DAW code is transmitted to the insurance company when the pharmacy bills for a prescription). The DAW code describes the factors that were taken into account when the pharmacist decided whether to dispense the generic form of the drug or the brand form.

DAW 0 = generic substitution permitted by prescriber
DAW 1 = generic substitution not allowed by prescriber
DAW 2 = generic substitution permitted, but patient requested brand product
DAW 3 = generic substitution permitted, but pharmacist selected brand
DAW 4 = generic substitution permitted, but generic not in-stock
DAW 5 = generic substitution permitted, but brand dispensed as generic
DAW 6 = all-purpose override
DAW 7 = law mandated that the brand product be dispensed
DAW 8 = generic substitution permitted, but generic not available on the market
DAW 9 = other

What is Wholesale Acquisition Cost (WAC)?
WAC is the price a wholesaler would pay a manufacturer to purchase a drug.

Why is WAC important?
WAC is commonly used when pricing drugs items.

Example Problems
What is the retail cost (cost to the customer) of Drug X if WAC is $49.56, the markup is 20%, and the dispensing fee is $10?
Retail Cost = WAC + Markup + Dispensing Fee
Retail Cost = $49.55 + ($49.56 x 0.2) + $10 = $69.46

What would the WAC be for Drug Y if the retail cost is $9.00, the dispensing fee is $2.00, and the markup is 25%?
WAC = Retail Cost – Dispensing Fee – Markup
WAC = $9.00 – $2.00 – ($7.00 x 0.25) = $5.60

Practice Problems
1. What is the retail cost of Drug B if WAC = $20, the dispensing fee = $8, and the markup is 50%?

2. What is the WAC of Drug C if the retail cost is $99.96, the markup is $15%, and the dispensing fee is $7.50?

Practice Problem Answers
1. $38
2. $80.40

Dosing Frequency

QOD = every other day

QD = each day (daily)

BID = twice daily

TID = three times daily

QID = four times daily

QAM = every morning

QPM = every evening

Qwk = every week

Qmo = every month

H = hours

D = days

^{o} = hours (e.g. Q6^{o} = every 6 hours)

hs = bedtime

ac = before meals

cf = with food

wf = with food

pc = after meals

WA = while awake

ATC = around the clock

NTE = not to exceed

PRN = as needed

STAT = immediately

Routes of Administration

PO = by mouth

PR = rectally

PV = vaginally

AU = both ears

AS = left ear

AD = right ear

OU = both eyes

OS = left eye

OD = right eye

IV = intravenous

IVP = intravenous push

IVPB = intravenous piggyback

IM = intramuscular

ID = intradermal

IC = intracardiac

IP = intraperitoneal

IN = intranasal

NG = nasogastric

SQ = subcutaneous

SL = sublingual (under the tongue)

TD = transdermal (across the skin)

Dosing Instructions

UD = as directed

AAA = apply to affected area

Dispensing Instructions

QS = sufficient quantity

NR = no refills

DAW = dispense as written (dispense brand only)

Compounding Instructions

aa = of each

div = divide

Symptoms and Disease States

N/V = nausea and vomiting

HBP = high blood pressure

HTN = hypertension

BPH = benign prostatic hyperplasia (enlarged prostate)

GAD = generalized anxiety disorder

SAD = seasonal effective disorder

CRC = colorectal cancer

Units of Measure

kg = kilogram (one thousand grams)
g = gram
mg = milligram (one one-thousandth of a gram)
μg = microgram (one one-millionth of a gram)
gr = grain (1 grain = 64.8 mg)
gtt = drop
gtts = drops
tsp = teaspoon (5 mL)
tbs = tablespoon (15 mL)
oz = ounce (one fluid ounce = 29.67 mL; one ounce of weight = 28.35 grams)
L = liter
mL = milliliter (one one-thousandth of a liter)
μL = microliter (one one-millionth of a liter)
M = molar
mM = millimolar
mEq = milliequivalent
IU = international unit

Formulations

cr = cream
crm = cream
oint = ointment
ung = ointment
lot = lotion
top = topical
inj = injection
tab = tablet
cap = capsule

susp = suspension
syr = syrup
supp = suppository
CR = controlled release
DR = delayed release
ER = extended release
LA = long acting
SR = sustained release
XR = entended release

Clean Room

PPE = personal protective equipment
D5W = 5% dextrose in water
D10W = 10% dextrose in water
NSS = normal saline solution = 0.9% sodium chloride in water
½ NS = one-half normal saline = 0.45% sodium chloride in water
D5NS = 5% dextrose in normal saline
RL = Ringer's Lactate
LR = Lactated Ringers
SWFI = sterile water for injection
LVP = large volume parenteral (infusion volume greater than 100 mL)
SVP = small volume parenteral (infusion volume equal to or less than 100 mL)
MVI = multivitamin
TPN = total parenteral nutrition

Miscellaneous

USP = United States Pharmacopoeia
NPO = nothing by mouth
D/C = discontinue
$\bar{c}$ = with
$\bar{s}$ = without
$\bar{ss}$ = one-half

NKA = no known allergies
NKDA = no known drug allergies
BP = blood pressure
IOP = intraocular pressure
HRT = hormone replacement therapy

Elements/Lab Values

Ca = calcium
Cl = chloride
Fe = iron
K = potassium

Mg = magnesium
Na = sodium
Phos = phosphate
Li = lithium

Practice Problems

1. Give $\bar{ss}$ tsp PO cf QID x 10D

2. Inj 12 units SQ QHS

3. Insert 1 supp PR Q6H PRN

4. 1 – 2 tabs PO Q4-6H PRN severe pain

5. 1 cap PO up to Q6H PRN N/V

6. AAA on face QPM HS

7. 1 tab PO QD for HTN

8. Inj 0.25 cc IM Qmo UD

9. Instill 1 gtt OS Q2H WA

Practice Problem Answers

1. Give one-half teaspoonful (2.5 mL) by mouth with food 4 times daily for 10 days.
2. Inject 12 units subcutaneously every night at bedtime.
3. Insert one suppository rectally every 6 hours as needed.
4. Take one to two tablets by mouth every 4 to 6 hours as needed for severe pain.
5. Take one capsule by mouth up to every 6 hours as needed for nausea and vomiting.
6. Apply to affected area on face every evening at bedtime.
7. Take one tablet by mouth once daily for hypertension.
8. Inject one-fourth mL (0.25 cc) intramuscularly every month as directed.
9. Instill one drop into left eye every two hours while awake.

APAP = Acetaminophen
ASA = Aspirin
CPZ = Chlorpromazine
DM = Dextromethorphan
EES = Erythromycin Ethylsuccinate
EPO = Erythropoietin
HC = Hydrocortisone
HCTZ = Hydrochlorothiazide
INH = Isoniazid
KCl = Potassium chloride
MgSO4 = Magnesium sulfate
MMI = Methimazole

MOM = Milk of Magnesia
MSO4 = Morphine sulfate
MTX = Methotrexate
NTG = Nitroglycerin
OC = Oral Contraceptive
PB = Phenobarbital
PCN = Penicillin
PE = Phenylephrine
PSE = Pseudoephedrine
PTU = Propylthiouracil
TAC = Triamcinolone
TCN = Tetracycline

Note: Though many prescribers still use them, it is generally best to avoid the use of abbreviations due to the potential for misinterpretation.

There are three systems of measurement used in pharmacy: the apothecaries' system, the avoirdupois system, and the metric system.

Apothecaries' System
The apothecaries' system was used in ancient Greece. For the most part, this measurement system is outdated, but a few older drugs do still express dosage strength in units of grains. Examples include: aspirin, ferrous sulfate, Armour Thyroid, nitroglycerin, and phenobarbital. In this system, the grain is the smallest unit of weight, and the minim is the smallest unit of volume.

Weight
1 grain (gr) = 64.8 milligrams
1 scruple (Ɔ) = 20 grains
1 dram (Ʒ) = 3 scruples
1 ounce (℥) = 8 drams
1 pound = 12 ounces

Volume
1 minim (♏) ~ 0.0617 mL
1 fluid dram = 60 minims
1 fluid ounce = 8 fluid drams
1 pint = 16 fluid ounces
1 quart = 2 pints
1 gallon = 4 quarts

Avoirdupois System
The avoirdupois measurement system is the customary system of weights and measures in the United States. In this system, one pound equals 16 ounces.

Weight
1 grain = 64.8 mg
1 ounce (oz) = 437.5 grains
1 pound lb) = 16 ounces

Volume
1 fluid ounce = 29.57 mL
1 cup = 8 fluid ounces
1 pint = 2 cups
1 quart = 2 pints
1 gallon = 4 quarts

Metric System
The metric system is the standard measurement system for pharmacy and medicine. As a base ten system, it is also the simplest measurement system.

Weight
1 milligram (mg) = 1,000 micrograms
1 gram (g) = 1,000 milligrams
1 kilogram (kg) = 1,000 grams

Volume
1 milliliter (mL) = 1 cm^3 (cc)
1 liter (L) = 1,000 milliliters
1 deciliter (dL) = 100 milliliters

Roman Numerals
I = 1
V = 5
X = 10
L=50
C=100
D=500
M=1,000

Rules

1) When Roman numerals are repeated, add them together.
   - Example: III = I + I + I = 3
2) When a smaller Roman numeral is written to the right of a larger Roman numeral, add it to the larger Roman numeral.
   - Example: VI = V + I = 6
3) When a smaller Roman numeral is written to the left of a larger Roman numeral, subtract it from the larger Roman numeral.
   - Example IX = X – I = 9
4) Avoid using more than three of the same Roman numeral in a sequence.
   - Example: ~~IIII = 4~~   IV = 4
5) When rule 2 and 3 are in conflict, use rule 3.
   - Example: ~~XIX = 21~~   XIX = 19

Examples

Roman numeral III = 3
Roman numeral IV = 4
Roman numeral XIX = 19

Practice Problems

Convert the following numbers to Roman numerals:

1. 120
2. 80
3. 30
4. 3750
5. 1200
6. 473
7. 15
8. 291

Convert the following Roman numerals to numbers:

9. CL
10. XC
11. LXV
12. XLVIII
13. MM
14. CCXL
15. CDLXXX
16. CCLVI

Practice Problem Answers

1. CXX
2. LXXX
3. XXX
4. MMMDCCL
5. MCC
6. CDLXXIII
7. XV
8. CCXCI
9. 150
10. 90
11. 65
12. 48
13. 2000
14. 240
15. 480
16. 256

There are three ways to express an average: Mean, Median, and Mode.

Mean – Add up all the values and divide by the number of values.
> *Example*
> Seven values are given: 1, 4, 6, 3, 9, 8, 3
> Add the seven values: $1 + 4 + 6 + 3 + 9 + 8 + 3 = 34$
> Divide by seven: $34 \div 7 = 4.9$
> Mean = 4.9

Median – Determine the middle number.
> *Example*
> Nine values are given: 11, 3, 10, 5, 4, 5, 5, 8, 7
> Rearrange values into chronological order: 3, 4, 5, 5, 5, 7, 8, 10, 11
> Determine the middle number: 3, 4, 5, 5, 5, 7, 8, 10, 11
> Median = 5

Mode – Identify the value that appears most often in a set of values.
> *Example*
> Eight values are given: 4, 6, 7, 1, 3, 1, 3, 1
> Tally the number of times each value is presented and identify the most commonly presented value:
> > 1: III
> > 3: II
> > 4: I
> > 6: I
> > 7: I
> Mode = 1

Example Problem
A patient measured her blood glucose level daily for one week. Based on her measurements, what was her mean blood glucose for the week?

Monday: 190 mg/dL
Tuesday: 182 mg/dL
Wednesday: 110 mg/dL
Thursday: 90 mg/dL
Friday: 125 mg/dL
Saturday: 130 mg/dL
Sunday: 70 mg/dL

Solution:

$$\frac{\left(190 + 182 + 110 + 90 + 125 + 130 + 70\right) \text{mg/dL}}{7} = 128 \text{ mg/dL}$$

Answer: 128 mg/dL

Practice Problems
1. What is the median in the following set of numbers: 19, 12, 49, 34, 101, 67, 1?

2. What is the mode in the following set of numbers: 4, 2, 1, 4, 5, 2, 4, 3, 2, 1, 2, 4, 2?

3. What is the mean in the following set of numbers: 3, 1, 4, 5, 2, 3, 5, 1, 5, 3, 2, 2, 4?

Practice Problem Answers
1. 34
2. 2
3. 3.1

Must-know Conversion Factors

1 ounce (weight) = 28.35 g
1 fluid ounce (volume) = 29.57 mL*
*Some pharmacists round up to 30 mL.

1 teaspoon (tsp) = 5 mL
1 tablespoon (tbs) = 3 teaspoons

1 Cup = 8 fluid ounces
1 Pint = 2 cups = 16 fluid ounces
1 Quart = 2 pints = 4 cups = 32 fluid ounces
1 Gallon = 8 pints = 4 quarts = 128 fluid ounces

1 gr = grain = 64.8 milligrams

1 gram = 1,000 milligrams
1 milligram = 1,000 micrograms

1 kg = 2.2 pounds

1 inch = 2.54 centimeters

The unit conversion/proportion approach is a *very* versatile problem solving tool. Many text books try to teach you a more complex version of this concept that is unnecessarily difficult. The approach I am about to teach you is the same one that I successfully use to solve nearly *all* of the problems I encounter in my everyday work. The best advice to mastering this approach is to do *a lot* of example and practice problems, plenty of which you will find in the following pages. This concept carries over into other sections as well, so you will get even more practice as you proceed through the book. Below is the general equation you will use:

$$(\text{\# in Given Units}) \times (\text{ConversionFactor*}) = \text{\# in Desired Units}$$
*Conversion Factor = Desired Units/Given Units

Example Problems
How many fluid ounces (℥) are in 118 mL (answer in Roman numerals)?

Solution:

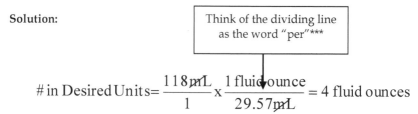

Think of the dividing line
as the word "per"***

$$\# \text{ in Desired Units} = \frac{118\,\text{mL}}{1} \times \frac{1 \text{ fluid ounce}}{29.57\,\text{mL}} = 4 \text{ fluid ounces}$$

<u>Note</u>: notice how the milliliter units cancel out.

Answer: IV ℥   (4 fluid ounces)

***There are 29.57 milliliters **per** fluid ounce (29.57 mL/fluid ounce). This can be written as "29.57 mL/1 fluid ounce" **or** "1 fluid ounce/29.57 mL." Since 1 fluid ounce is *equal* to 29.57 mL, then 29.57 mL ÷ 1 fluid ounce = 1.

Multiplying a value by the factor "29.57 mL/1 fluid ounce" is like multiplying it by 1. The actual value doesn't change, but the units do change. This is true when you multiply any number by a conversion factor.

Since multiplying by the factor "29.57 mL/1 fluid ounce" is mathematically the same as multiplying by 1, then multiplying the reciprocal "1 fluid ounce/29.57 mL" is also like multiplying by 1. How do you know which way to orient the conversion factor? You have to decide which units you want on top (the numerator) and which units you want on the bottom (the denominator) based on what units you are trying to obtain. The units you are trying to obtain should go on top (numerator) and the units you are trying to eliminate should go on the bottom. See below for an example of what happens when you orient the conversion factor *the wrong way*:

$$\frac{118\,\text{mL}}{1} \times \frac{29.57\,\text{mL}}{1 \text{ fluid ounce}} = 3,489.26\,\text{mL}^2/\text{fluid ounce}$$

Clearly this did **not** give us the units we desired.

How many kilograms (kg) does a 77 lb patient weigh?

Solution:

$$\# \text{ in Desired Units} = \frac{77\,\text{lb}}{1} \times \frac{1\,\text{kg}}{2.2\,\text{lb}} = 35\,\text{kg}$$

Answer: 35 kg

How many milliliters are in 16 ounces?

Solution:

$$\# \text{ in Desired Units} = 16 \text{ ounces} \times \frac{29.57 \text{ mL}}{\text{ounce}} = 473 \text{ mL}$$

Note: milliliters (mL) are the Desired Units, because we want to know the # of mL in 16 ounces. Likewise, the # in Given Units is 16 ounces, as that is the value we were given. Since we know the conversion factor (29.57 mL per ounce), we have all the information needed to solve the problem.

Answer: 473 mL

A patient drops off a prescription for 30 tablets of 5 grain ferrous sulfate. You only have four iron products stocked in the pharmacy. Which of the four products should you dispense?
A. Fergon® (Ferrous gluconate 250 mg)
B. Ferro-Sequels® (Ferrous fumarate 150 mg)
C. Feosol® (Ferrous sulfate 325 mg)
D. SlowFe® (Ferrous sulfate 225 mg)

Solution:

$$\# \text{ in Desired Units} = \frac{5 \text{ grains}}{1} \times \frac{64.8 \text{mg}}{\text{grain}} = 324 \text{mg}$$

Answer: C. Feosol® (Ferrous sulfate 325 mg)

You receive a prescription order for Nitrostat® sublingual tablets 1/200 grain. Nitrostat® sublingual tablets are available in 3 strengths. Which strength should you dispense?
A. 0.3 mg
B. 0.4 mg
C. 0.6 mg

Solution:

$$\# \text{ in Desired Units} = \frac{1 \text{ grain}}{200} \times \frac{64.8 \text{mg}}{\text{grain}} = 0.3 \text{mg}$$

Answer: A. 0.3 mg

An order comes to the pharmacy for levothyroxine 0.125 mg IV injection. Using a levothyroxine 40 mcg/mL solution, how many milliliters should you dispense?

    A. 0.0031 mL

    B. 3.1 mL

    C. 0.31 mL

    D. 3.1 µL

Solution:

$$\# \text{ in Desired Units} = \frac{0.125\,\text{mg}}{1} \times \frac{1,000\,\mu\text{g}}{\text{mg}} \times \frac{\text{mL}}{40\,\mu\text{g}} = 3.1\,\text{mL}$$

Answer: B. 3.1 mL

A patient weighs 100.1 kg. What is the patient's weight in pounds?

Solution:

$$\# \text{ in Desired Units} = \frac{100.1\,\text{kg}}{1} \times \frac{2.2\,\text{lb}}{1\,\text{kg}} = 220\,\text{lb}$$

Answer: 220 lb

The Glucagon Emergency Kit for Low Blood Sugar, manufactured by Lilly, comes with a vial containing 1 mg of glucagon and 49 mg of lactose. Assuming Lilly has all the glucagon it needs, how many vials can they prepare using only one pound of lactose?

$$\frac{1\,\text{pound lactose}}{1} \times \frac{16\,\text{oz.}}{\text{pound}} \times \frac{28.35\,\text{g}}{\text{oz.}} \times \frac{1,000\,\text{mg}}{\text{g}} = 453,600\,\text{mg lactose}$$

$$\frac{453,600\,\text{mg lactose}}{1} \times \frac{\text{vial}}{49\,\text{mg lactose}} = 9,257.14\,\text{vials}$$

Answer: 9,257 vials

Sometime the conversion factor will be hidden in the words. Take this problem for example: What is the days' supply of a bottle of 90 tablets of levothyroxine 112 mcg if the instructions are to take one tablet by mouth every day, except take one-half tablet on Sundays?

Solution:

$$\frac{90 \text{ tablets}}{1} \times \frac{7 \text{ days}}{6.5 \text{ tablets}} = 96 \text{ days}$$

Note: The conversion factor here was 6.5 tablets/7 days.

Answer: 96 days

Given a solution that contains 100 mg of drug per 5 mL, how many milliliters would be required to obtain a dose of 650 mg?

Solution:

$$\frac{650 \text{ mg}}{1} \times \frac{5 \text{ mL}}{100 \text{ mg}} = 32.5 \text{ mL}$$

Answer: 32.5 mL

Sometimes, you will need to do a series of conversions to reach the answer you need. Take this problem for example: How many 75 mcg tablets can be made from six pounds of a drug?

Solution:

$$\frac{6 \text{ pounds}}{1} \times \frac{16 \text{ ounce}}{\text{pound}} \times \frac{28.35 \text{ g}}{\text{ounce}} \times \frac{1,000,000 \text{ mcg}}{\text{g}} \times \frac{\text{tablet}}{75 \text{ mcg}}$$

$$= 36,288,000 \text{ tablets}$$

Answer: 36,288,000 tablets

Practice Problems

1. How many fluid ounces are in a jug containing 3,785 mL of polyethylene glycol with electrolytes?

2. After reconstitution, how many teaspoons are in three 100-mL bottles of Amoxicillin 250 mg/5 mL oral suspension? Express your answer in Roman numerals.

3. Approximately how many tablespoons are in a 4 oz bottle of cough syrup?

4. How many scruples of aspirin are in sixteen 5 grain tablets of Ecotrin®?

5. If a patient is 6 feet tall, how tall would the patient be in centimeters?

6. You have 7 pounds of triamcinolone 0.1% ointment. How many kilograms do you have?

7. How many tablespoons are in a 150-mL bottle of an antibiotic suspension?

8. How many milliliters of a 200 mg/mL solution of testosterone cypionate should be injected intramuscularly if the patient needs to receive 75 mg per injection?

9. How many milliliters are needed to provide one 300 mg dose of amoxicillin using a 250 mg/5 mL amoxicillin suspension?

10. A patient applied 4 g of Voltaren® 1% Gel (10 mg diclofenac/1 g gel) to her knee. How many milligrams of diclofenac were applied to her knee?

11. A physician wrote a prescription for testosterone cypionate 200 mg/mL solution with the instructions to inject 0.75 mL intramuscularly once every two weeks. How many grams of the drug will the patient inject over the course of one year?

Practice Problem Answers
1. 128 fluid ounces
2. LX teaspoons
3. 8 tablespoons
4. 4 scruples
5. 183 centimeters
6. 3.18 kilograms
7. 10 tablespoons
8. 0.375 milliliters
9. 6 mL
10. 40 mg
11. 3.9 g

When insurance companies are billed for prescriptions, the pharmacy technician and pharmacist are responsible for entering the correct days' supply being dispensed. If you bill an insurance company for a days' supply less than that actually dispensed (e.g. bill a 30-day supply of medication as though it was a 10-day supply) the insurance company can issue a "charge-back" during an audit (i.e. the pharmacy would have to pay the insurance company back). Most prescriptions are dispensed for tablets or capsules (i.e. solid oral dosage forms). In these cases, determining the days' supply is a simple one-step calculation.

Example Problems
What is the days' supply for a prescription of 30 tablets of Drug X with the instructions to take one tablet by mouth once daily?

$$\frac{30 \text{ tablets}}{1} \times \frac{\text{day}}{1 \text{ tablet}} = 30 \text{ days}$$

What is the days' supply for a prescription of 60 tablets of Drug AB9012 with the instructions to take one tablet three times daily as needed for pain?

$$\frac{60 \text{ tablets}}{1} \times \frac{\text{day}}{3 \text{ tablets}} = 20 \text{ days}$$

Note: When the instructions include the term "as needed," assume the patient will use the maximum amount when calculating the days' supply.

Calculating the days' supply of a non-solid dosage form (e.g. oral liquids, eye drops, ear drops, nasal sprays, and inhalers) can be more challenging. Review the example problems below, then practice it yourself until you master it!

When necessary, use this information to complete the problems in this section:
ProAir®, Proventil®, and Ventolin® all contain 120 puffs/inhaler
Astepro® nasal spray contains 200 sprays/bottle
Flonase® nasal spray contains 120 sprays/bottle
Xalatan® eye drops contain 2.5 mL/bottle

More Example Problems

How many days will a 4-ounce bottle of cetirizine 5 mg/5 mL solution last if the instructions are to take one-half teaspoonful QHS?

$$\frac{120\,mL}{bottle} \times \frac{tsp}{5\,mL} \times \frac{day}{0.5\,tsp} = 48\,days/bottle$$

What would the days' supply be on a prescription for Flonase® nasal spray if the instructions are 1 spray in each nostril QD?

$$\frac{120\,sprays}{bottle} \times \frac{day}{2\,sprays} = 60\,days/bottle$$

Calculate the days' supply of 1 bottle of Astepro® with the instructions to spray 1 spray in each nostril BID.

Days' supply = 50 days

A prescription is written for 3 Ventolin® HFA Inhalers with the instructions to inhale 2 puffs PO Q4-6H PRN wheezing. Each inhaler contains enough medication for 200 puffs. What would the days' supply of this prescription be?

$$\frac{3\,inhalers}{1} \times \frac{200\,puffs}{inhaler} \times \frac{day}{12\,puffs} = 50\,days$$

Prednisone is available in 5 mg and 10 mg dose packs. These dose packs are available in quantities sufficient to last how many days?

Two sizes are available for each strength: a 48 tablet 6-day dose pack & a 21 tablet 12-day dose pack.

****

Test Your Knowledge
How many drops are there in one milliliter?
15 – 20 drops.

<u>Note</u>: In general, you should calculate days' supply based on 20 drops/mL, but when answering multiple choice questions you should calculate days' supply based on 15 drops/mL and 20 drops/mL. This way you know the answer is one of the two or somewhere in between. See below for example.

****

What is the days' supply for a 7.5 mL bottle of Ciprodex® Otic Solution with the instructions: ii gtts AS QID until gone?

    A.   7 days
    B.   10 days
    C.   14 days
    D.   20 days
    E.   25 days

Solution:

Step 1: *Interpret the sig.*

"ii gtts AS QID until gone"
= Place two drops into the left ear four times daily until gone.

Step 2: *Since the question does not specify how many drops are in one milliliter, calculate the days' supply based on 15 drops/mL **and** 20 drops/mL.*

$$\frac{7.5\ mL}{1} \times \frac{15\ drops}{mL} \times \frac{day}{8\ drops} = 14\ days$$

$$\frac{7.5\ mL}{1} \times \frac{20\ drops}{mL} \times \frac{day}{8\ drops} = 18\ days$$

Answer: C. 14 days
Note: If you only calculated the days' supply based on 20 drops/mL, you likely would have rounded up to 20 days' supply and missed this one.

You are dispensing a 5-mL bottle of ciprofloxacin 0.3% ophthalmic solution with instructions to instill two drops into each eye three times daily until gone. What is the days' supply of this prescription (assume 20 drops/mL)?

$$\frac{5\ mL}{1} \times \frac{20\ drops}{mL} \times \frac{day}{12\ drops} = 8\ days$$

****
The Rule of Hand
One (1) gram of topical medication is roughly enough to cover one side (palm and fingers) of four flat hands. Use the Rule of Hand when calculating the days' supply of topical medications.
****

Practice Problems

1. What is the days' supply for a 15-gram tube of acne medication with instructions to apply to the entire face nightly?
Note: The area of the face is roughly equal to the area of two flat hands.

2. You are dispensing two Ventolin® HFA inhalers with instructions for the patient to inhale one to two puffs by mouth every four to six hours as needed for shortness of breath. What will the days' supply be for this prescription?

3. What is the days' supply for a quantity of 60 venlafaxine ER 37.5 mg capsules with the following instructions: i PO QD x 7 days, then i PO BID x 7 days, then ii QAM and i QPM thereafter?

4. What is the days' supply for a 120-mL bottle of Tussionex® suspension with the following instructions: take i tsp PO up to TID PRN for cough?

5. A prescription for methotrexate 2.5 mg tablets has the instructions to take three tablets by mouth weekly. How long will a prescription for 30 tablets last?

6. NovoLog FlexPen is available in a package that contains five pens. Each pen holds three mL of NovoLog insulin. If a patient uses 11 units SQ every morning and 9 units SQ every evening with a meal, what is the days' supply for one package?

7. Antipyrine and benzocaine otic solution comes in a 15-mL bottle. What is the days' supply if the instructions are as follows: instill 2-4 gtts AU up to QID PRN?
Note: Assume there are 20 drops per mL.

Practice Problem Answers
1. 30 days
2. 33 days
3. 27 days
4. 8 days
5. 70 days
6. 75 days
7. 9 days

Density (δ) = mass (grams) per unit volume (milliliters).

$$\text{Density} = \frac{\text{Mass}}{\text{Volume}}$$

Specific gravity = density of a substance relative to the density of a reference substance*.

$$\text{Specific Gravity} = \frac{\text{Density of Substance}}{\text{Density of Reference Substance}}$$

*The reference substance is almost always H_2O (water), which has a density of 1 g/mL. When this is the case, the specific gravity of a substance is the same value as the density, just without the units. For example, the density of glycerin is 1.26 g/mL. When you calculate the specific gravity of glycerin, you take the density of glycerin and divide it by the density of water (1.26 g/mL ÷ 1 g/mL = 1.26). Essentially all that happens is the units cancel out, and you get specific gravity of glycerin = 1.26.

Example Problems
You weigh 30 mL of a substance to determine what it is. If the substance weighs 33.3 grams, what is the identity of the substance?

        A. Water (density = 1. 0 g/mL)
        B. Isopropyl Alcohol (density = 0.79 g/mL)
        C. Glycerin (density = 1.26 g/mL)
        D. Simple Syrup (density = 1.3 g/mL)
        E. Ethylene Glycol (density = 1.11 g/mL)

Solution:

$$\text{Density} = \frac{\text{Mass}}{\text{Volume}}$$

$$\text{Density} = \frac{33.3\,\text{g}}{30\,\text{mL}} = 1.11\,\text{g/mL}$$

Answer: E. Ethylene Glycol (Density = 1.11 g/mL)

To compound a 60 gram formulation that contains 10% (w/w) petrolatum, how many milliliters of pure hot liquid petrolatum would be required?
Note: Density of petrolatum = 0.9 g/mL

Solution:

$$\frac{10\,\text{g petrolatum}}{100\,\text{g total}} \times \frac{60\,\text{g total formulation}}{1} = 6\,\text{g petrolatum}$$

$$\frac{6\,\text{g petrolatum}}{1} \times \frac{\text{mL}}{0.9\,\text{g}} = 6.67\,\text{mL petrolatum}$$

Answer: 6.67 mL of petrolatum

Practice Problems

1. How much does 4 mL of a substance weigh if its density is 1.2 g/mL?

2. What volume of simple syrup (density 1.3 g/mL) would be needed to obtain a 2 gram sample?

3. What would the specific gravity of water be (density = 1 g/mL) if the reference substance was glycerin (density = 1.26 g/mL)?

4. If 78 mL of Substance H weighs 131 grams, what is the density of Substance H?

5. If 12 grams of Liquid Q has a volume of 15 mL, what is the specific gravity of Liquid Q (assume reference substance is water)?

Practice Problem Answers
1. 4.8 g
2. 1.54 mL
3. 0.79
4. 1.68 g/mL
5. 0.8

A temperature conversion problem will be easy points on the PTCB exam if you know how to solve it. Memorize the equations for converting Fahrenheit to Celsius and Celsius to Fahrenheit and know how to apply them.

Converting from **Fahrenheit to Celsius:**

$$^\circ C = \frac{5}{9}(^\circ F - 32)$$

Converting from **Celsius to Fahrenheit:**

$$^\circ F = \left(\frac{9}{5} \times {}^\circ C\right) + 32$$

****

Temperature Conversion Values to Memorize
0°C = 32°F (freezing point of water)
37°C = 98.6°F (human body temperature)
100°C = 212°F (boiling point of water)

****

Example Problem
You read that insulin should be stored at 2 – 8°C. What is this temperature range in degrees Fahrenheit?

Solution:

$$\left(\frac{9}{5} \times 2^\circ C\right) + 32 = 36^\circ F \qquad \left(\frac{9}{5} \times 8^\circ C\right) + 32 = 46^\circ F$$

Answer: 36 – 46°F

Practice Problems
Convert the following temperature to degrees Fahrenheit:

1) –3°C
2) 0°C
3) 1°C
4) 6°C
5) 25°C
6) 60°C

Convert the following temperatures to degrees Celsius:

7) –10°F
8) 0°F
9) 32°F
10) 98.6°F
11) 72°F
12) 101°F

Practice Problem Answers
1) 27°F
2) 32°F
3) 34°F
4) 43°F
5) 77°F
6) 140°F
7) -23°C
8) -18°C
9) 0°C
10) 37°C
11) 22°C
12) 38.3°C

Weight-based dosing always requires the patient's weight to be in units of kilograms (kg). Some problems you encounter may simply involve converting a weight in pounds to a weight in kilograms. However, it is more likely that converting a patient's weight from units of pounds to kilograms will be the first step in a multi-step calculation. Because there are so many problems that could begin with converting weight from pounds to kilograms, it is extremely important that you master this calculation. How can you master this calculation? It is simple, just remember that 1 kg = 2.2 lbs, and then do example and practice problems until this calculation is second nature for you.

Infliximab is prescribed to a patient at the dose of 5 mg/kg. The patient weighs 154 pounds. How many milligrams of infliximab should be in one dose?

$$\frac{154\,pounds}{1} \times \frac{1\,kg}{2.2\,pounds} \times \frac{5\,mg}{kg} = 350\,mg$$

You calculate the appropriate dose of infliximab to be 350 mg. The dose is going to be administered IV in 250 mL of 0.9% NaCl. Infliximab comes in a vial containing 100 mg/20 mL solution. How many vials will you need to open in order to fill this prescription?

4 vials.

How many milliliters of the drug solution will you need in order to obtain the 350 mg of infliximab to fill the aforementioned prescription?

$$\frac{350\,mg}{1} \times \frac{20\,mL}{100\,mg} = 70\,mL$$

Vancomycin is being dosed at 15 mg/kg for a patient that weighs 241 pounds and has a fever. How many milliliters of vancomycin 1 gram/20 mL solution will be needed to compound this prescription?

$$\frac{241\,pounds}{1} \times \frac{1\,kg}{2.2\,pounds} \times \frac{15\,mg}{kg} \times \frac{20\,mL}{1\,g} \times \frac{1\,g}{1,000\,mg} = 32.9\,mL$$

Note: Frequently you will receive problems that contain irrelevant information (in this case, the fact that the patient has a fever). Don't be distracted by this type of information, just move on and solve the problem.

Formula for Body Surface Area (BSA):

$$\sqrt{\frac{\text{height}(\text{cm})\text{x weight (kg)}}{3,600}}$$

What drugs are commonly dosed by body surface area (BSA)?
Cancer chemotherapy drugs.

What is the BSA of a patient that is 5 feet and 4 inches tall and weighs 110 pounds?

$$\sqrt{\frac{64\,\text{inches}}{1}\text{x}\frac{2.54\,\text{cm}}{\text{inch}}\text{x}\frac{110\,\text{lbs}}{1}\text{x}\frac{1\,\text{kg}}{2.2\,\text{lbs}}\text{x}\frac{1}{3,600}}=1.50\,\text{m}^2$$

Note: BSA is expressed in square meters (m²).

The appropriate dose of Doxorubicin is 550 mg/m2. How many milligrams are required to provide three doses to a male patient 6′ 1″ tall weighing 225 lbs?

$$\frac{73\,\text{inches}}{1}\text{x}\frac{2.54\,\text{cm}}{\text{inch}}=185\,\text{cm}\qquad\frac{225\,\text{lbs}}{1}\text{x}\frac{1\,\text{kg}}{2.2\,\text{lbs}}=102\,\text{kg}$$

$$\left(\sqrt{\frac{185\,\text{cm x}102\,\text{kg}}{3600}}\right)\text{x}\frac{550\,\text{mg}}{\text{m}^2}\text{x}\frac{3\,\text{doses}}{1}=3777\,\text{mg}$$

Note: When you convert the height and weight to the metric system separately (as was done above) and then plug the numbers into the equation for BSA, your final answer will be slightly less accurate due to rounding. For this reason, it is better to calculate your height and weight and plug the values in all in one step (see below for example).

$$\left(\sqrt{\frac{73\,\text{in}}{1}\text{x}\frac{2.54\,\text{cm}}{\text{in}}\text{x}\frac{225\,\text{lb}}{1}\text{x}\frac{1\,\text{kg}}{2.2\,\text{lb}}\text{x}\frac{1}{3600}}\right)\text{x}\frac{550\,\text{mg}}{\text{m}^2}\text{x}\frac{3}{1}=3787\,\text{mg}$$

This answer is more accurate, since the converted weight and height were not rounded.
In this case, there were only 2 significant figures, so technically, the correct answer is 3,800 mg. So both approaches yield the same answer for all practical purposes; however, it is always best to use the most accurate approach when solving math problems and then round your final answer up or down as necessary.

The key to solving drip rate problems is figuring out the volume (i.e. the number of milliliters) that needs to be infused into the patient over a specified period of time (e.g. each minute). Once you know the volume that needs to be infused per unit time, all you need to do is convert the volume from milliliters to drops based on how many drops per milliliter the administration set delivers (e.g. a microdrip administration set delivers 60 drops/mL). Then you will have your answer. It is simple unit conversion – take the given information and convert the units until you get the drip rate (drops/minute).

Test Your Knowledge
How many drops are there in one milliliter?
15-20 drops.

Some IV administration sets deliver 60 drops/mL, what are these called?
Microdrip administration sets.

Example Problems
A 500 mL solution contains 2 grams of Drug X. How many mL/minute should be administered for the patient to receive 200 mg/hour?

Solution:
Step 1: *Determine the concentration of infusion solution.*

$$\frac{2 \text{ grams}}{1} \times \frac{1{,}000 \text{mg}}{\text{gram}} \times \frac{1}{500 \text{mL}} = 4 \text{ mg/mL}$$

Step 2: *Calculate the infusion rate in units of mL/min.*

$$\frac{200 \text{mg}}{\text{hr}} \times \frac{\text{mL}}{4 \text{ mg}} \times \frac{\text{hr}}{60 \text{min}} = 0.83 \text{mL/min}$$

Answer: 0.83 mL/min

In the problem above, what would the drip rate be assuming a drip set delivering 60 drops/mL is being utilized?

Solution:

$$\frac{0.83 \text{ mL}}{\text{min}} \times \frac{60 \text{ drops}}{\text{mL}} = 49.8 \text{ drops/min} \sim 50 \text{ drops/min}$$

Answer: 50 drops/min

A patient is receiving 15,000 units of heparin per hour from an IV bag containing 250 mL of 100 unit/mL heparin. If the administration set delivers 20 drops/mL, how many drops is the patient receiving each minute?

Solution:

$$\frac{15,000\,\cancel{units}}{\cancel{hr}} \times \frac{\cancel{mL}}{100\,\cancel{units}} \times \frac{20\,drops}{\cancel{mL}} \times \frac{\cancel{hr}}{60\,min} = 50\,drops/min$$

Note: Don't forget, you must be able to recognize when certain information is irrelevant (e.g. the fact that the bag is 250 mL is an irrelevant piece of information).

Answer: 50 drops/min

Milrinone is being dosed at 0.33 mcg/kg/min for a 210 lb patient with a creatinine clearance of 30 mL/min. The infusion bag contains Milrinone 40 mg in 200 mL of D5W. What is the drip rate if a microdrip administration set (60 drops/min) is being used?

Solution:

$$\frac{0.33\,\cancel{mcg}}{\cancel{kg} \bullet min} \times \frac{210\,\cancel{lb}}{1} \times \frac{\cancel{kg}}{2.2\,\cancel{lb}} \times \frac{200\,\cancel{mL}}{40\,\cancel{mg}} \times \frac{1\,\cancel{mg}}{1,000\,\cancel{mcg}} \times \frac{60\,drops}{\cancel{mL}} = 9\,drops/m$$

Answer: 9 drops/min

A physician orders Vasopressin 30 milliunits/min. You dispense a 250-mL sterile admixture containing 25 units of Vasopressin in normal saline. What should the drip rate be if the administration set delivers 20 drops per minute?

Solution:

$$\frac{30\,\cancel{milliunits}}{min} \times \frac{250\,\cancel{mL}}{25\,\cancel{units}} \times \frac{\cancel{unit}}{1,000\,\cancel{milliunits}} \times \frac{20\,drops}{\cancel{mL}} = 6\,drops/min$$

Answer: 6 drops/min

Practice Problems

1. What is the drip rate for a 250-mL bag of Vancomycin 1g in NSS if it is infused over one hour using a microdrip administration set (60 drops/milliliter)?

2. An administration set delivering 30 drops/mL was used to infuse a 160-mL bag of magnesium sulfate solution over the course of 120 minutes. What was the drip rate?

3. Drug M is available as a 100 mcg/1 mL infusion. If the patient receiving this infusion weighs 176 pounds and Drug M is being dosed at 10 mcg/kg/hr, what should the drip rate be using a microdrip administration set?

4. A patient receives 1 liter of Drug P over 24 hours. What is the drip rate using an administration set that delivers 19 drops/mL?

Practice Problem Answers
1. 250 drops/minute
2. 40 drops/minute
3. 8 drops/minute
4. 13 drops/minute

What are the three major methods for calculating pediatric doses based on adult dosing information?

1. Clark's Rule
2. Young's Rule
3. BSA dosing

Clark's Rule

$$Child\,Dose = \frac{Child's\ Weight\,(lbs)}{150\,lbs} \times Adult\,Dose$$

What is the significance of the value 150 lbs?
150 lbs is the average adult weight.

Young's Rule

$$Child\,Dose = \frac{Child's\ Age}{(Child's\ Age + 12)} \times Adult\,Dose$$

BSA Dosing

$$Child\,Dose = \frac{Child's\ BSA}{1.73m^2} \times Adult\,Dose$$

What is the significance of the value 1.73 m²?
1.73 m² is the average adult body surface area (BSA).

Example Problems
You are dispensing a prescription for prednisone for a 6-year-old patient that is
3′ 5″ tall and weighs 49 pounds. What is the appropriate pediatric dose for this
patient based on BSA dosing if the adult dose is 20 mg?

Solution:

$$\text{Child Dose} = \frac{\sqrt{\dfrac{\dfrac{41\,\text{in}}{1} \times \dfrac{2.54\,\text{cm}}{\text{in}} \times \dfrac{49\,\text{lbs}}{1} \times \dfrac{\text{kg}}{2.2\,\text{lbs}}}{3,600}}}{1.73\,\text{m}^2} \times 20\,\text{mg} = 9.3\,\text{mg}$$

Answer: 9.3 mg

What is the appropriate dose based on Young's Rule?

Solution:

$$\text{Child Dose} = \frac{6}{(6+12)} \times 20\,\text{mg} = 6.7\,\text{mg}$$

Answer: 6.7 mg

What is the appropriate dose based on Clark's Rule?

Solution:

$$\text{Child Dose} = \frac{49\,\text{lbs}}{150\,\text{lbs}} \times 20\,\text{mg} = 6.5\,\text{mg}$$

Answer: 6.5 mg

Using Clark's Rule, calculate the appropriate dose of Drug X for a 30 kg child (the adult dose is 750 mg).

    A.   150 mg
    B.   250 mg
    C.   300 mg
    D.   330 mg
    E.   460 mg

Solution:

$$\text{Child Dose} = \frac{\left(\dfrac{30\,kg}{1} \times \dfrac{2.2\,lbs}{kg} \right)}{150\,lbs} \times 750\,mg = 330\,mg$$

Answer: D. 330 mg

<u>Note</u>: Never overlook what units you are working with. If you forgot to convert the patient's weight from kilograms to pounds, you would have missed this question.

Practice Problems

1. The adult dose of Drug HD3021 is 400 mg once daily. What is the appropriate dose of Drug HD3021 for a 10-year-old male child that is 53 inches tall and weighs 78 pounds? Use Clark's Rule.

2. The adult dose of a drug is 150 mg twice daily for three days. How many milligrams (for a three-day course of therapy) should be dispensed to an 8-year-old female child that is 45 inches tall and weighs 57 pounds? Use Young's Rule.

3. Based on an adult dose of 600 mg, what is the appropriate dose for a 6-year-old boy that is 3 feet 4 inches tall and weighs 44 pounds? Use BSA Dosing.

4. If the adult dose if a drug is 1 gram, what is the appropriate dose for an 11-year-old child that weighs 100 pounds? Use Clark's Rule.

5. If the adult dose if a drug is 1 gram, what is the appropriate dose for an 11-year-old child that weighs 100 pounds? Use Young's Rule.

Practice Problem Answers

    1.   208 mg
    2.   360 mg (60 mg per dose x 6 doses)
    3.   260 mg
    4.   667 mg
    5.   478 mg

The human body naturally produces steroid hormones. Taking steroids medicinally causes a reduction in the body's steroid production. At high doses, use of medicinal steroids can shut down steroid hormone production within the body. For this reason, when high doses of medicinal steroids are discontinued, it is necessary to decrease the dose gradually over time (as opposed to abruptly stopping the medication) to give the body the time it needs to turn steroid production back on. The process of gradually reducing the dose of a steroid is called a steroid taper.

Often steroids are tapered through the use of a dosepak. An example of a steroid dosepak is the prednisone 10 mg 6-day dosepak where the patient takes 6 tablets the first day and decreases by one tablet daily until finished (6, 5, 4, 3, 2, 1, stop). With dosepaks, the instructions are included in the packaging, so prescribers will often provide the instructions "UD" (take as directed).

It should be noted that steroid taper regimens do not always come in a dosepak. In these cases, the prescriber will write out the specific instructions. For example, take 30 mg daily for 3 days, 20 mg daily for 3 days, 10 mg daily for 3 days, 5 mg daily for 3 days, and then stop.

> Note: "taper" is a term that also applies to gradually increasing the dose of a medication. Upward tapers are most commonly seen with anticonvulsants and medications used to treat psychiatric conditions.

When dealing with tapers, days' supply calculations can be complicated, but it is important that they are done correctly. Remember, when an insurance company is improperly billed for a prescription, they can recoup their money in an audit (the pharmacy must pay them back). For instance, if an insurance company audits your pharmacy and finds that a prescription is dispensed for a 21 days' supply, but the insurance is billed as though the prescription was a 10 days' supply, the insurance company can refuse to pay the pharmacy for the prescription and the pharmacy loses that money.

Weight/Weight % (w/w) = # of grams of API* per 100 grams of preparation.
Example
AndroGel® 1% gel contains 1 g testosterone per 100 grams of gel.

Practice Problem
How many milligrams of testosterone are contained in one 5-gram packet of AndroGel® 1% gel?

$$\frac{1\,g\ testosterone}{100\,g\,gel} \times \frac{5\,g\,gel}{1} \times \frac{1,000mg}{g} = 50\,mg\,testosterone$$

Weight/Volume % (w/v) = # of grams of API* per 100 mL of preparation.
Example
Clindamycin 1% topical solution contains 1 g clindamycin per 100 mL of solution.

Practice Problem
What is the percent concentration (w/v) of a 250-mL solution that contains 35 mg of an active ingredient?

$$\frac{0.035g}{250mL} = \frac{x}{100mL} \quad \therefore \quad x = \frac{0.035g \times 100mL}{250mL} = 0.014g$$

$$0.014g/100mL = 0.014\%\,(w/v)$$

Volume/Volume % (v/v) = # of mL of API* per 100 mL of preparation.
Example
Charatussin® AC contains 3.8% (v/v) alcohol, meaning that it contains 3.8-mL of alcohol in every 100-mL of Cheratussin® AC solution.

Practice Problem
What is the percent concentration (v/v) of a 15-mL bottle of a solution that contains 0.75-mL tea tree oil in sterile water?

$$\frac{0.75mL\,API}{15\,mL} = \frac{x}{100mL} \quad \therefore \quad x = \frac{0.75mL\,API \times 100mL}{15\,mL} = 5\,mL$$

$$5\,mL/100mL = 5\%\,(v/v)$$

*API = active pharmaceutical ingredient

When expressing a concentration as a percent, why is it necessary to specify whether the concentration is in terms of w/w, w/v, or v/v?

It is necessary to specify because some substances can only be measured feasibly by weight (i.e. solid substances) and some substances are easier to measure by volume (i.e. liquids). Weight and volume are not equal (e.g. 1 mL of alcohol weighs 0.79 grams), except in the case of water (1 mL of water weighs 1 gram). This is because different substances have different densities (see section titled "Density and Specific Gravity" for more details on density).

More Practice Problems

1. A 6-month-old female is given one-half dropperful of Sodium Fluoride 0.11% (w/v) drops. How many milligrams of Sodium Fluoride did she receive?
Note: 1 dropperful = 1 mL

2. Clobetasol propionate topical solution comes in a 50-mL bottle. If each mL of solution contains 0.5 mg of clobetasol propionate, what is the percent concentration of the solution?

3. Prednisolone 15 mg/5 mL oral solution contains 5% (v/v) alcohol. How many milliliters of alcohol are there in one teaspoonful of solution?

4. Antipyrine and benzocaine otic solution contains 1.4% (w/v) benzocaine and 5.4% (w/v) antipyrine in an anhydrous glycerin base. How many milligrams of each active ingredient are present in one 15-mL bottle?

Practice Problem Answers
1. 0.55 mg Sodium Fluoride
2. 0.05% (w/v)
3. 0.25 mL alcohol
4. 810 mg of antipyrine & 210 mg of benzocaine

Ratios are used in:
1. Compounding recipes.
2. Expressing the concentration of a medication.

Ratios Used in Compounding Recipes
When used in a compounding recipe, ratios function to describe how many parts of each substance make up the whole. For instance, a 24-ounce cherry pie recipe that calls for a 1:1 ratio of pie dough to cherry filling would be comprised of 12 ounces of pie dough and 12 ounces of cherry filling.

When compounding a medication, you will be given three pieces of information.
1. The ingredient names.
2. The amount of each product to add relative to the other (i.e. the ratio).
3. The amount of final product desired.*

* In some cases, the amount of final product desired may be written by the prescriber as "QS" which is from the Latin phrase "quantum sufficit" meaning "as much as suffices." In these cases, you will need to calculate how much to prepare based on the dosing instructions. See **Example Problem** below.

Example Problems
How much of each ingredient would be needed to compound the following prescription?

1:2 mixture of Lidocaine 2% & Diphenhydramine 12.5 mg/5 mL
Dispense Quantity: QS
Sig: swish and swallow 3 teaspoonsful PO QID x 14 days
Refills: 0 (no refills)

Solution:

Step 1: *Since the quantity is written as QS, you must calculate the amount of final product desired. This is easy, because you know how much product is being used in one dose (3 teaspoonsful), you know how many doses the patient will take each day (4 doses/day), and you know how long the patient will be taking the medication (14 days).*

$$\frac{15\,\text{mL}}{\text{dose}}\times\frac{4\,\text{doses}}{\text{day}}\times\frac{14\,\text{days}}{1}=840\,\text{mL}$$

Step 2: *Calculate the amount that makes up 1 part of the 3 part mixture by dividing the amount of final product desired by 3 parts.*

$$\frac{840\,\text{mL}}{3\,\text{parts}} = 280\,\text{mL/part}$$

Step 3: *Now that you know the amount that represents 1 part, calculate the amount of each ingredient that will be needed to compound the prescription.*

$$\frac{1\,\text{part Lidocaine2\%}}{1} \times \frac{280\,\text{mL}}{\text{part}} = 280\,\text{mL Lidocaine2\%}$$

$$\frac{2\,\text{parts Diphen.12.5mg/5mL}}{1} \times \frac{280\,\text{mL}}{\text{part}} = 560\,\text{mL Diphen.12.5mg/5mI}$$

Answer: 280 mL Lidocaine 2% & 560 mL diphenhydramine 12.5 mg/5 mL

Ratios Used to Express the Concentration of a Medication

When used to express a concentration, a ratio functions to describe how many parts of the active ingredient are present in a certain number of parts of the total formulation. For example, epinephrine 1:10,000 solution contains one part epinephrine in 10,000 parts of solution. Remember the conversion factors below for your reference.

Conversion Factors for Concentrations Expressed by a Ratio
1:1 = 1 x 10⁰ grams per 1 mL = 1 g/mL
1:1,000 = 1 x 10⁻³ grams per 1 mL = 1 mg/mL
1:1,000,000 = 1 x 10⁻⁶ grams per 1 mL = 1 mcg/mL

Example Problem

How many mg of epinephrine are there in 2 mL of Epinephrine 1:1,000,000 solution?

Solution:

Step 1: *Convert the ratio into a value with metric units using the conversion factor above.*

According to conversion factor above, 1:1,000,000 = 1 mcg/mL.

Step 2: *Apply the following equation or use the unit conversion/proportion approach.*

$$\frac{\text{Weight}_1}{\text{Volume}_1} = \frac{\text{Weight}_2}{\text{Volume}_2}$$

Insert the given information into the equation.

Weigth$_1$ = 1 mcg
Volume$_1$ = 1 mL
Weight$_2$ = ?
Volume$_2$ = 2 mL

$$\frac{1 \text{ mcg}}{1 \text{ mL}} = \frac{\text{Weight}}{2 \text{ mL}}$$

Step 3: *Get the unknown value (Weight$_2$) alone.*

$$\text{Weight} = \frac{1 \text{ mcg} \times 2 \text{ mL}}{1 \text{ mL}} = 2 \text{ mcg}$$

Answer: 2 mcg

Practice Problems

1. The package for EpiPen Jr 2-Pak® comes with 2 Auto-Injectors, each one containing 0.3 mL of a 1:2000 epinephrine solution. How many milligrams of epinephrine are in one EpiPen Jr 2-Pak®?

2. What is the ratio strength of a 20-mL solution that contains 200 mcg of drug?

3. What is the ratio strength of a solution that contains 1 mg of drug per mL of solution?

4. How many milliliters of a 1:200 stock solution of Lidocaine would be required to compound a prescription for 50 mL of 0.25% Lidocaine solution?

5. If you have 1 gallon of a 1:40 solution of Drug XYZ, how many Liters of 1:1,000 solution of Drug XYZ can you compound?

Practice Problem Answers

1. 0.3 mg (0.15 mg of epinephrine per Auto-Injector, and there are two Auto-Injectors in one EpiPen Jr 2-Pak®)
2. 1:10,000
3. 1:1,000
4. 25 mL
5. 94.6 L

Alligation is a great way to solve certain compounding math problems. Use alligation when you are given two products with different concentrations of the same drug and you need a concentration that falls somewhere in the between (or when you have a higher concentration than what is desired and you want to dilute it with an inert substance like water or petrolatum). Start by drawing an X with a hollow center.

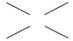

In every alligation problem, you will have to compound a prescription for a certain concentration using two products. One product will have a higher-than-desired concentration, and the other product will have a lower-than-desired concentration. As an example, lets say we have a 1% cream of Product B and a 10% cream of Product B, and we want to make a cream that contains 3% Product B. Write the value for the high concentration product at the top left of the hollow X, and write the value for the low concentration product at the bottom left of the hollow X.

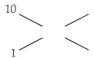

Next, write the value of the desired concentration in the center of the hollow X.

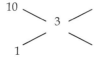

Then calculate the difference between the numbers on the left side of the X and the number at the center of the X. Write the answer, following the diagonal line, at the opposite corner of the X.

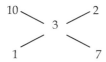

The numbers on the right side of the X indicate the proportion of each ingredient that will be needed to compound a formulation of the desired concentration.

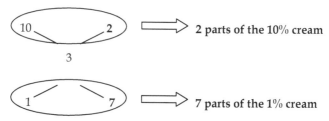

10   2   ⟹   **2 parts of the 10% cream**

     3

1   7   ⟹   **7 parts of the 1% cream**

At this point, you would have all the information needed to solve the problem. Let's say the prescription called for 60 grams of 3% Product B cream. Based on the results of the alligation, you know that the cream would be made up of nine equal parts (2 parts of 10% cream and 7 parts of 1% cream). Divide 60 grams into nine equal parts (60 g ÷ 9 parts = 6.67 g/part). You would need 13.3 g (6.67 g/part x 2 parts = 13.3 g) of 10% cream and 46.7 g (6.67 g/part x 7 parts = 46.7 g) of 1% cream to compound 60 g of 3 % Product B cream. Now, practice as many of these as you can!

Practice Problems
You need 30 g of Triamcinolone 0.05% ointment, but all you have in stock is Triamcinolone 0.025% and 0.1% ointment. How much of each ingredient will you need in order to compound this prescription?

Solution:

0.1   0.025

       0.05

0.025   0.05

$$0.025 : 0.05 = 1 : 2$$

1 part 0.1% triamcinolone : 2 parts 0.025% triamcinolone

$$\frac{30\,g}{3\,parts} \times \frac{1\,part\,0.1\%\,triamcinolone}{1} = 10\,g\,0.1\%\,triamcinolone$$

$$\frac{30\,g}{3\,parts} \times \frac{2\,parts\,0.025\%\,triamcinolone}{1} = 20\,g\,0.025\%\,triamcinolone$$

Answer: 10 g of 0.1% and 20 g of 0.025% triamcinolone ointment

You have 800 mL of 70% alcohol solution. How much water will you need to add in order to make a 10% alcohol solution?
Note: Assume the water contains 0% alcohol.

Solution:

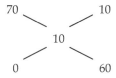

$$10\,\text{parts} = 800\,\text{mL} \therefore 1\,\text{part} = 80\,\text{mL}$$

$$60\,\text{parts} \times \frac{80\,\text{mL}}{\text{part}} = 4{,}800\,\text{mL}$$

Answer: 4,800 mL of water

How many grams of pure Sodium Chloride must be added to 10 mL of normal saline solution to create a 3% NaCl solution?
Note: Pure NaCl is 100% NaCl.

Solution:

$$\begin{array}{ccc} 0.9 & & 97 \\ & 3 & \\ 100 & & 2.1 \end{array}$$

$$97\ \text{parts of } 0.9\%\ \text{NaCl} = 10\ \text{mL} \therefore 1\ \text{part} = \frac{10\ \text{mL}}{97} = 0.103\ \text{mL}$$

$$2.1\,\text{parts} \times \frac{0.103\text{mL}}{\text{part}} = 0.22\,\text{mL} \sim 0.22\text{g}$$

Answer: 0.22 g of pure NaCl

You need to compound an IV solution of 2.5 mg/mL Vancomycin in D5W using a vial that contains 1 gram of Vancomycin in 20 mL. How much D5W will be needed?

Solution:

<u>Step 1</u>: *Convert the concentrations to percentages.*

> Note: A one-percent solution contains one gram per one hundred milliliters (1% = 1 g/100 mL). Given this fact, you can convert the given units to a percentage by calculating the number of grams in 100 mL.

$$\frac{2.5\,mg}{mL} \times \frac{g}{1,000\,mg} \times 100 = 0.25g/100\,mL = 0.25\%$$

$$\frac{1\,g}{20\,mL} \times 5 = 5\,g/100\,mL = 5\%$$

> To summarize, we are given a 5% Vancomycin solution, a 0% Vancomycin solution (D5W), and we want to create a 0.25% Vancomycin solution.

<u>Step 2</u>: *Alligation math.*

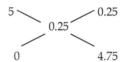

$$0.25\,parts\,5\%\,vancomycin\,4.75\,parts\,D5W$$

In other words (if you multiply each part by a factor of 4), the compound must be made up of 1 part of 5% Vancomycin and 19 parts D5W.

We know we are using 20 mL of the 5% Vancomycin solution, so:

$$1\,part = 20\,mL \therefore 19\,parts = 19 \times 20\,mL = 380\,mL$$

Answer: 380 mL of D5W

Practice Problems

1. How much of each ingredient will be needed to make 50 mL of 1% KCl solution from 3% KCl solution and water?

2. How many Liters of 3% H_2O_2 and 6% H_2O_2 will you need to mix together to make 2 Liters of 4.5% H_2O_2?

3. You need to dilute a 5% Lidocaine cream to compound 45 grams of 4% Lidocaine cream using a cream base. How much 5% Lidocaine cream will be needed to compound this prescription?

4. How many grams of 1% Hydrocortisone cream will need to be mixed with 100% Hydrocortisone powder to make 2 ounces of 2.5% Hydrocortisone cream?
Note: 1 ounce = 28.35 grams

Practice Problem Answers

1. 16.7 mL of 3% KCl solution; 33.3 mL of water
2. 1 Liter of 3% H_2O_2 & 1 Liter of 6% H_2O_2
3. 36 grams of 5% Lidocaine cream
4. 55.8 grams of 1% Hydrocortisone cream

What does the term "aseptic" mean?
Without organisms (i.e. sterile).

What is a beyond use date (BUD)?
A beyond use date is the date after which a compounded medication should not be used. Beyond use dates are typically short (i.e. days, weeks, or months) compared to expiration dates which are usually one or more years. This is because the long-term stability of compounded medications is usually unknown.

True or false. A beyond use date and an expiration date are the same thing.
False, manufacturers assign expiration dates to manufactured products, whereas beyond use dates are assigned to compounded drug products.

What is the most common cause of contamination?
Touch contamination (i.e. the sterile product is contaminated by contact with skin of the hand).

When washing your hands prior to preparing a compounded sterile product (CSP), what should you use?
A. Antibacterial soap and hot water.
B. Antibacterial soap and warm water.
C. Antibacterial soap and cold water.

> **Answer:**
> B. Antibacterial soap and warm water.

What is the proper procedure for hand washing prior to entering the clean room?
Wash the hands and arms all the way up to the elbows vigorously for at least 30 seconds paying special attention to the fingernails and the spaces between the fingers.

What is the technical term for a pharmacy clean room?
Buffer area.

What chapter of the United States Pharmacopoeia (USP) is concerned with compounded sterile products?
USP Chapter 797.

What is the ultimate goal of USP Chapter 797?
To protect patients from receiving contaminated infusions.

According to USP Chapter 797, what cosmetics and accessories cannot be worn in the buffer area?
- Makeup
- Jewelry
- Watches
- Nail polish
- Artificial nails

Does USP Chapter 797 permit eating and/or drinking in the buffer area?
No.

There are 5 levels of risk associated with compounded sterile products. What are the risk levels and how are they defined?

1. <u>Immediate-use category</u>
- Prepared using aseptic technique, but not in a clean room environment.
- Takes less than 1 hour to compound the formulation.
- Can be administered within 1 hour of compounding.
- Only for emergency situations where low-risk compounding procedures would lead to an unreasonable delay in therapy.
  - BUD 1 hour (refrigeration or room temperature)

2. <u>Low-risk level</u>
- Prepared using aseptic technique in a clean room environment.*
- Simple admixtures (up to 3 ingredients added with 2 entries into the infusion bag) using closed system transfer methods.
- Ingredients are sterile.
  - BUD 48 hours (room temperature)
  - BUD 14 days (refrigeration)
  - BUD 45 days (frozen at a temperature = or < 10°C)

3. <u>Low-risk level with < 12 hour BUD</u>
- Prepared in an ISO Class 5 LAFH outside of a clean room environment (i.e. not inside a buffer area with an ante room).
- Simple admixtures (up to 3 ingredients added with 2 entries into the infusion bag) using closed system transfer methods.
- Ingredients are sterile.
- Must be administered within 12 hours of being prepared.
  - BUD 12 hours (refrigeration or room temperature)

4. <u>Medium-risk level</u>
- Prepared using aseptic technique in a clean room environment.
- Complex manipulations (several ingredients and entries into the bag) or extensive amount of time required to compound (e.g. TPN preparations, batch compounded preparations).
- Formulations that are to be used over several days.
- Ingredients are sterile.
  - BUD 30 hours (room temperature)
  - BUD 9 days (refrigeration)
  - BUD 45 days (frozen at a temperature = or < 10°C)

5. <u>High-risk level</u>
- Prepared in a clean room environment.
- Ingredients are not sterile (e.g. bulk powders), or compounding method involves open system transfers.
- Improper garb.
  - BUD 24 hours (room temperature)
  - BUD 3 days (refrigeration)
  - BUD 45 days (frozen at a temperature = or < 10°C)

*A *clean room environment* means in an ISO Class 5 LAFH located within an ISO Class 7 buffer area adjacent to an ISO Class 8 ante area.

The principles of sterile compounding are referred to as _____.
Aseptic technique.

What type of container must be used for the disposal of needles?
A red sharps container.

Sterile alcohol swabs are soaked in what type of alcohol?
70% isopropyl alcohol.

What is the purpose of a laminar airflow hood (LAFH)?
To create an environment with a very low concentration of particles and microorganisms in the air so that formulations safe enough for human infusion can be prepared.
    Note: LAFH may be abbreviated as LAFW (laminar airflow workbench).

How many air filters is a LAFH equipped with?
2 air filters (1 regular filter and 1 HEPA filter).

What is a HEPA filter?
HEPA stands for "High Efficiency Particulate Air." HEPA filters remove 99.97% of particles from the air that are 0.3 microns (micrometers) or larger.

How frequently should you wipe or spray a HEPA filter with alcohol?
Never, this would damage the filter membrane.

A LAFH must be turned on for how many minutes prior to use?
30 minutes.

Besides being turned on for 30 minutes, what else must be done prior to using a LAFH?
It must be cleaned with 70% isopropyl alcohol.

How frequently should a LAFH be cleaned with alcohol when in constant use?
Every 30 minutes.

To assure that filtered air is reaching the critical site, you must work at least __ inches inside the LAFH.
6.

In a LAFH, you want to avoid placing your hands or other objects behind the materials you are working with because you want to prevent _____.
Airflow obstruction.

What type of hood should be used to compound chemotherapy infusions?
A biological safety cabinet.

Vials have a rubber stopper. If the medication contained in a vial would undergo a chemical reaction with rubber, what type of container could the manufacturer use instead?
An ampule (which is an all-glass container).

Infusion filters are available with many different pore sizes. Smaller pore sizes filter out more unwanted particles, but are more prone to clogging. What are some examples of unwanted particles that filters are helpful in removing?
Glass particles, rubber fragments, dust, clothing fibers, fungi, and bacteria.

What is a micron?
A micron is a measure of length equal to one one-millionth of one meter.

What pore size is optimal for removing microorganisms, such as bacteria and fungi?
0.22 μm (referred to as a "0.22 micron filter").

What is total parenteral nutrition?
Nutrients delivered via intravenous route for the purpose of bypassing the gastrointestinal tract.

What is the difference between a TPN (total parenteral nutrition) and a TNA (total nutrition admixture)?
A TPN is a 2-in-1 mixture of amino acids and dextrose (plus electrolytes), whereas a TNA is a 3-in-1 mixture which includes the above plus a fat (lipid) component.

> Note: frequently you will hear people refer to a TNA as a TPN (as though they are synonymous), even though *technically* they are not the same type of preparation.

What would happen if you used a 0.22 micron filter on a TNA (3-in-1)?
The filter would get clogged by the fat component of the TNA.

What is the optimal pore size for filtering an infusion that contains fat (as is found in a TNA infusion)?
1.2 microns (1.2 μm).

What are the benefits and drawbacks of a 1.2 micron filter?
BENEFITS:
- Good flow of emulsified fat and other contents through the filter.
- Low probability of clogging.
- Fungi are filtered out.

DRAWBACK:
- Some bacteria and other materials smaller than 1.2 microns are not filtered out.

What is the most important compatibility consideration in TNA preparation?
The incompatibility between calcium and phosphate. If the concentration of these two ions is too high, an insoluble precipitate will form in the TNA. TNAs contain fat which turns the mixture white and opaque, making it nearly impossible to see calcium phosphate precipitates.

When compounding a TPN or TNA, how can you minimize the risk of calcium phosphate precipitate formation?
By adding phosphate toward the beginning of the compounding process and adding calcium last.

What issue must be considered when including insulin in a TPN or TNA?
Up to 50% of the insulin will bind to the surface of the inside of the bag and administration system (tubing).

What can happen when vitamin C (ascorbic acid) is included in a TPN or TNA?
Over time, ascorbic acid degrades to oxalic acid, which forms an insoluble precipitate with calcium called calcium oxalate.

Why are we concerned about precipitate formation?
Precipitates are solid particles. If a solid particle is infused into a patient's bloodstream, it can get stuck in a blood vessel and block the flow of blood. This can lead to a cardiovascular event (e.g. heart attack, stroke, pulmonary embolism).

Many vials say "single-dose" on the label, indicating that the contents are preservative-free. Once the stopper of a single-dose vial is punctured, in what time frame must you to use the contents of the vial?
- If the vial is stored in less than ISO Class 5 air, you have 1 hour to use it.
- If stored in ISO Class 5 or cleaner air, you have 6 hours to use it.

True or false. Needles and syringes are sterile inside their packaging.
True.

Anatomy of a Needle

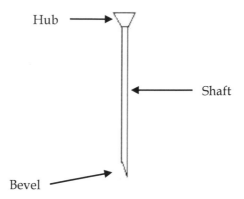

Hub

Shaft

Bevel

Understanding Needle Gauges

30 Gauge Needle   16 Gauge Needle

<u>Key point</u>: Gauge is inversely proportional to the diameter of the needle lumen. In other words, the higher the gauge, the smaller the hole the needle will make.

Can the syringe pictured below be used to accurately measure 11 mL? Why or why not?

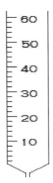

Yes, syringes measure accurately up to one-half of the smallest marked unit. Since the syringe pictured above contains markings for every 2 mL, it can be used to accurately measure to the nearest 1 mL. However, a 20-mL syringe would be better suited to measure 11 mL.

When mixing medications for IV administration, it is important to look for signs of incompatibility. What are some common signs of incompatibility?
- Gas formation (bubbles)
- Precipitate formation (solid particles)
- Turbidity (cloudiness)
- Color change

What is a diluent?
A diluent is an inactive product used to dilute an active pharmaceutical ingredient.

What is trituration?
Trituration is the process of reducing the particle size of a powder, usually by use of a mortar and pestle.

What is a class A prescription balance?
A class A prescription balance is the standard balance used by pharmacists when compounding medications.

What is "sensitivity requirement?"
The sensitivity requirement is the mass needed to move the balance marker by one space (see below for an illustration). For a class A prescription balance, the sensitivity requirement is 6 mg.

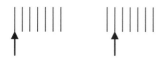

What is geometric dilution?
Geometric dilution is the process of expanding the weight of the active pharmaceutical ingredient by adding an inert substance (i.e. diluent) in a fashion that yields a homogenous mixture.

What is the purpose of geometric dilution?
Many drug doses are very small (in the microgram to milligram range). Accurately measuring these small doses can be difficult. To obtain an accurate measurement, you have two options: 1) use a highly sensitive analytical balance or 2) dilute the drug to make its mass larger. The standard pharmacy balance is a class A prescription balance. This type of balance is sensitive enough to measure 120 mg of more within 5% error. To accurately measure smaller quantities, you have to dilute the drug.

For example
If you want to measure 60 mg of a drug using a class A prescription balance, you could take 120 mg (the lowest quantity that can be accurately measured) of the pure (100%) drug powder and mix it with 120 mg of lactose (an inert substance; diluent). Now you have a powder that is 50% drug and 50% lactose. Now you can measure 120 mg of the mixture to obtain 60 mg of drug. The trick is to never use the balance to measure any quantity less than 120 mg. If you do, you will not be within the 5% error requirement (to gain a better understanding of percent error, refer to page 71).

How do you perform geometric dilution?

Take the active pharmaceutical ingredient and add an equal amount of diluent. Triturate the mixture until you are convinced it is homogenous. Then add an equal amount of diluent to the mixture and triturate as before. Repeat the steps until all of the ingredients have been mixed together.

Illustrated Example of Geometric Dilution

Dilute 200 mg of amlodipine powder with 1,400 mg of lactose powder to create a 1,600 mg homogenous mixture containing 200 mg of amlodipine.

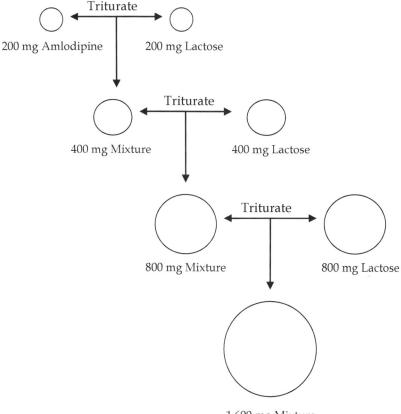

1,600 mg Mixture
(200 mg Amlodipine & 1,400 mg Lactose)

<u>Key Point</u>: If you just triturate 200 mg of amlodipine with 1,400 mg of lactose all in one step, you would probably achieve an uneven (heterogeneous) mixture. By slowly adding the diluent, as is done in geometric dilution, you greatly increase the likelihood of achieving an even (homogenous) mixture.

What is the percent error (% error)?

Percent error refers to the accuracy of a measurement. For instance, 5% error means that the measurement is within +/- 5% of the actual value. In pharmacy, the highest acceptable percent error is 5%, and can be even less in some cases (e.g. narrow therapeutic index or highly potent drugs).

How are the "sensitivity requirement" and "percent error" related?

These terms are related according to the following equation:

$$\% \text{ Error} = \frac{\text{Sensitivity Requirement}}{\text{Desired Weight}} \times 100\%$$

Given that the sensitivity requirement of a class A prescription balance is 6 mg, what is the minimum quantity that can be weighed within 5% error?

Solution:

This problem can be solved using the above equation. The terms were re-written to reflect the nature of this specific question.

Note: LWQ = least weighable quantity.

$$\text{Maximum Acceptable \% Error} = \frac{\text{Sensitivity Requirement}}{\text{LWQ}} \times 100\%$$

$$5\% = \frac{6 \text{ mg}}{\text{LWQ}} \times 100\%$$

Rearrange the equation to get LWQ alone.

$$\therefore \text{ LWQ} = \frac{6 \text{ mg}}{5\%} \times 100\% = 120 \text{ mg}$$

Answer: 120 mg

If you were using a class A prescription balance to measure 20 mg of Powder X, what would the percent error be?

Solution:

$$\% \ Error = \frac{Sensitivity \ Requirement}{Desired \ Weight} \times 100\% = \frac{6 \ mg}{20 \ mg} \times 100\% = 30\%$$

Answer: 30% error

Is this an acceptable level of error?
No, the highest acceptable level of error is 5%.

If you needed to measure 20 mg of a Powder X using a class A prescription balance, how would you do it while achieving a percent error < or = 5%?
Take 120 mg of the substance (which can be measured with 5% error) and use geometric dilution to create a homogenous mixture of 1 part (120 mg) Powder X and 5 parts (600 mg) diluent (e.g. lactose). Then, using the class A prescription balance, measure out 120 mg of the mixture, which will contain 20 mg of Powder X.

You are compounding a prescription which requires you to measure 40 mL of a liquid. Which of the following pieces of equipment should you use?
   A.   10 mL graduated cylinder
   B.   50 ml graduated cylinder
   C.   20 mL syringe
   D.   60 mL syringe
   E.   1 mL pipette

Answer:
B. 50 mL graduated cylinder

****
Equipment Selection Tip
Use the smallest piece of equipment that will hold the desired volume.
****

Practice Problems

1. You want to measure 10 mg of a substance within 1% error without diluting it. The sensitivity requirement of your balance would need to be ___.

2. You are using a class A prescription balance to measure 9 grams of maltose. What percent error will you get with this measurement?

3. You want to measure out 20 mg of hydrocortisone with 5% error using a class A prescription balance. Since the LWQ (least weighable quantity) is 120 mg, you know you will have to perform a geometric dilution to obtain a 20 mg measurement within 5% error. How much diluent powder and hydrocortisone will need to be combined to perform the geometric dilution?

4. After completing the geometric dilution from *practice problem 3* (above), what is the ratio of hydrocortisone to diluent powder?

5. From *practice problem 3*, what is the percent concentration of hydrocortisone in the resulting powder mixture?

6. From *practice problem 3*, what is the fraction of hydrocortisone in the resulting powder mixture?

Practice Problem Answers

1) 0.1 mg
2) 0.067%
3) 600 mg of diluent powder & 120 mg of hydrocortisone
4) 1:5 hydrocortisone to diluent powder
5) 16.67%
6) 1/6

For people without vitamin deficiencies, the best source of vitamins is a well-balanced diet of wholesome foods. There are 4 fat-soluble vitamins: A, D, E, and K. All other vitamins are water-soluble. As a general rule, excessive doses of fat-soluble vitamins (A, D, E, and K) over a long period of time will lead to toxicity and adverse effects since they accumulate in fat tissue. On the other hand, excessively high doses of water-soluble vitamins are eliminated in the urine, and generally do not cause as many problems. However, keep in mind that excessively high doses of some water-soluble vitamins are still capable of producing adverse effects (e.g. diarrhea with vitamin C).

Vitamin A (Retinol)

Uses: Needed for low-light vision.

Recommended adult dose: 2,000 – 3,000 IU/day

Max dose: 10,000 IU/day; excessive doses in pregnant women can cause birth defects.

Notes: When beta-carotene is consumed, found in carrots and sweet potatoes, it gets converted to vitamin A inside the body.

Vitamin B1 (Thiamine)

Uses: Needed for metabolism of carbohydrates.

Recommended adult dose: 1 – 1.5 mg/day (10 mg/day for cataract prevention)

Max dose: None established.

Vitamin B2 (Riboflavin)

Uses: Needed for metabolism of fats, proteins, and carbohydrates.

Recommended adult dose: 1 mg/day

Max dose: None established.

Vitamin B3 (Niacin)

Uses: Lowers cholesterol and triglycerides.

Recommended adult dose: 14 – 18 mg/day

Max dose: 35 mg/day; excessive doses cause flushing.

Notes: Flushing can be prevented by taking an NSAID (e.g. aspirin) with the niacin.

Vitamin B5 (Pantothenic Acid)

Uses: Needed for metabolism of nutrients and synthesis of certain enzymes.

Recommended adult dose: 5 mg/day

Max Dose: None established; however, excessive doses can cause diarrhea.

Vitamin B6 (Pyridoxine)
Uses: Needed for metabolism, immune function, and fetal brain development.
Recommended adult dose: 1.5 mg/day
Max dose: 100 mg for adults; excessively high doses can cause severe nerve damage.

Vitamin B7 (Biotin)
Uses: Needed for metabolism of nutrients; commonly used to help strengthen nails and hair.
Recommended adult dose: 30 mcg/day.
Max dose: None established.

Vitamin B9 (Folic Acid)
Uses: Needed for cell development; most notably used during pregnancy to prevent fetal neural tube defects.
Recommended adult dose: 400 mcg/day (600 mcg/day for pregnant women)
Max dose: 1,000 mcg/day (higher doses may be used for certain conditions).

Vitamin B12 (Cobalamin)
Uses: Needed for DNA and red blood cell production.
Recommended adult dose: ~ 2.4 mcg/day
Max dose: None established (high doses have not been shown to be harmful).
Notes: A protein in the stomach called "intrinsic factor" is needed to absorb vitamin B12. Patients deficient in this protein become deficient in vitamin B12 and develop a condition known as "pernicious anemia." Like other types of anemia, this condition is characterized by a low red blood cell count. *Metformin* is a diabetes drug notorious for interfering with the body's ability to absorb vitamin B12.

Vitamin C (Ascorbic Acid)
Uses: Needed for its antioxidant properties to protect cells from free radical damage; the body also uses vitamin C in collagen production, which is needed for wound healing.
Recommended adult dose: 75 – 100 mg/day
Max dose: 2,000 mg/day; excessive doses can cause diarrhea and iron overload.
Notes: Vitamin C deficiency causes scurvy. Taking vitamin C with an iron supplement will increase the intestinal absorption of iron.

Vitamin D (Ergocalciferol (D2), Cholecalciferol (D3))

Uses: Needed for nerve function, immune function, and most notably for the absorption of dietary calcium.

Recommended adult dose: 400 – 800 IU/day

Max dose: 4,000 IU/day; excessive doses can damage kidneys and/or cause high calcium levels leading cardiac arrhythmias.

Notes: Vitamin D deficiency causes rickets in children and osteomalacia in adults, conditions in which the bones become brittle and soft. *Xenical®* *(orlistat) and Alli® (orlistat)* are weight-loss drugs that work by reducing intestinal absorption of fats. As a result, these drugs can lead to a deficiency in fat-soluble vitamins (A, D, E, and K).

Vitamin E (Alpha-tocopherol and 7 other related compounds)

Uses: Needed for its antioxidant properties to protect cells from free radical damage; the body also needs vitamin E for immune function and cardiovascular health.

Recommended adult dose: 22 IU/day

Max dose: 1,100 – 1,500 IU/day; excessive doses can cause bleeding.

Notes: Vitamin E deficiency is rare, but can cause nerve damage, muscle damage, and a weakened immune system. The risk for experiencing the side effect of bleeding while on vitamin E is especially high for patients on antiplatelet or anticoagulant medications like *aspirin, warfarin,* and *heparin.*

****

A note about antioxidants

Antioxidants tend to interfere with cancer chemotherapy and radiation, thus reducing the effectiveness of these cancer treatments. Why? Because antioxidants protect cells (including cancer cells) from free radicals, and often times free radicals (such as radiation) are used in an effort to kill cancer cells.

****

Vitamin K (Phytonadione)

Uses: Essential for blood clot formation; sometimes used topically to treat rosacea, stretch marks, scars, and burns; most notably used to reverse the effects of high doses of warfarin.

Recommended dose: 90 – 120 mcg/day

Max dose: None established.

Notes: Vitamin K intake should be consistent for patients using warfarin. If a patient ingests more than their normal amount of vitamin K while on warfarin, he/she would be at a higher risk for blood clots. If a patient ingests below their normal amount of vitamin K while on warfarin, he/she would be at a higher risk for bleeding.

Aloe *Used for burns/wounds (topical); Used to promote digestive health (oral)*

Biotin *Used to strengthen hair and nails*

Black Cohosh *Alleviates symptoms of menopause*

Cinnamon *Decreases blood sugar in diabetes*

Coenzyme Q-10 *Cardiovascular health*

Echinacea *Common cold prevention; Immune system booster*

Evening Primrose Oil *Skin disorders (topical); Menopause symptoms (oral)*

Feverfew *Treats migraine headaches*

Fish Oil *Used for cardiovascular health; Decreases triglyceride levels in the blood*

Flaxseed Oil *Used to reduce inflammation in arthritis and lower cholesterol*

Folic Acid *Taken before & during pregnancy to prevent fetal neural tube defects*

Garlic *Proven to decrease blood pressure*

Ginger *Treats nausea*

Gingko *Used to improve memory and increase blood circulation*

Glucosamine & Chondroitin *Used for joint pain/osteoarthritis*

Green Tea *Increases metabolism; Cancer prevention (antioxidant properties)*

Hoodia *Used to promote weight-loss*

Kava Kava *Used to treat anxiety*

Melatonin *Promotes sleep, used in treatment of insomnia*

Milk Thistle *Promotes liver health*

Peppermint *Used to treat heartburn and upset stomach*

Probiotics *Promotes digestive health; Replaces good bacteria killed by antibiotics*

Red Yeast Rice *Used to lower cholesterol*

St. John's Wort *Used to treat depression, has *many* drug interactions*

SAM-e *Used as a mood stabilizer*

Saw Palmetto *Used to treat BPH (enlarged prostate)*

Senna *Stimulant laxative*

Valerian *Used to treat insomnia and anxiety*

Witch Hazel *Used topically in the treatment of various skin conditions*

Yohimbe *Used for erectile dysfunction (can raise blood pressure excessively)*

OTC Pain Medications
Tylenol® (acetaminophen) *Fever, arthritis, headaches, and other aches/pains*
Excedrin® Migraine (acetaminophen, aspirin, caffeine) *Migraine headaches*
Ecotrin® (aspirin) *Fever, pain, blood clot prevention*
Advil®, Motrin® (ibuprofen) *NSAID – fever, inflammation, pain*
Aleve® (naproxen) *NSAID – fever, inflammation, pain*
Azo® (phenazopyridine) *Urinary pain*

OTC Antacids
Maalox® (aluminum hydroxide/magnesium hydroxide/simethicone)
Heartburn/Gas

OTC Laxatives
Metamucil® (psyllium fiber) *Constipation*
Citrate of Magnesium (magnesium citrate) *Constipation*
Milk of Magnesia® (magnesium hydroxide) *Constipation, heart burn*
Colace®, Senokot® (docusate) *Mild constipation*
Senokot-S® (docusate/sennosides) *Constipation, opioid-induced constipation*
Dulcolax® (bisacodyl) *Constipation, colonoscopy preparation*
Miralax® (polyethylene glycol (PEG) 3350) *Constipation, colonoscopy
preparation*

OTC Cough and Cold Medications
Delsym® (dextromethorphan) *Antitussive (suppresses cough)*
Robitussin® (guaifenesin) *Expectorant (thins mucus)*
Sudafed® (pseudoephedrine) *Decongestant (reduces sinus congestion)*

OTC Allergy Medications (Antihistamines)
Benadryl® *Allergies/allergic reactions*
Claritin® *Allergies*
Zyrtec® *Allergies*
Alavert® *Allergies*
Allegra® *Allergies*
Afrin® *Nasal allergies (nasal spray)*
Zaditor® (ketotifen) *Allergic conjunctivitis (eye drop)*

OTC Jock Itch, Athlete's Foot, and Ringworm Medications (Antifungals)
Lamisil® (terbinafine)
Lamisil® AF (tolnaftate)
Lotrimin® (clotrimazole)
Zeasorb® (miconazole)

The top 235 prescription drugs are listed. Included is the brand name of the drug (if applicable), the generic name in parenthesis, the available strengths, and the route of administration. To interpret abbreviations, refer to the *Abbreviation Legend* below. Drugs are grouped by primary indication (e.g. pain, anxiety, cough). To prepare for the PTCB exam, focus on brand & generic names and primary indications.

Abbreviation Legend:
PO – oral tablet or capsule
SC – subcutaneous injection
IV – intravenous injection
IM – intramuscular injection
ER – extended release
LA – long acting
DR – delayed released
CR – controlled release
C-II – Schedule II controlled substance
C-III – Schedule III controlled substance
C-IV – Schedule IV controlled substance
C-V – Schedule V controlled substance

Underactive Thyroid (Hypothyroidism)
Synthroid®, Levoxyl® (levothyroxine)
25, 50, 75, 88, 100, 112, 125, 137, 150, 175, 200, 300 mcg (PO)

Low Potassium (Hypokalemia)
K-Dur®, Klor-Con® (potassium chloride)
8, 10, 15, 20 mEq (PO)

Weight Loss
Adipex-P® (phentermine) *C-IV*
37.5 mg (PO)

Osteoporosis Treatment/Prevention
Actonel® (risedronate)
5, 30, 35, 150 mg (PO)

Boniva® (ibandronate)
150 mg (PO)
1 mg/mL solution (IV)

Fosamax® (alendronate)
5, 10, 35, 70 mg (PO)
70 mg/75mL (oral solution)

Evista® (raloxifene) *also used for prevention of breast cancer*
60 mg (PO)

Malaria
Qualaquin® (quinine)
324 mg (PO)

Anxiety
Xanax® (alprazolam) *C-IV*
0.25, 0.5, 1, 2 mg (PO)
Note: Xanax® XR is an extended-release tablet available in 0.5, 1, 2, and 3 mg strengths.

Ativan® (lorazepam) *C-IV*
0.5, 1, 2 mg (PO)
2 mg/mL, 4 mg/mL (IV solution)

Klonopin® (clonazepam) *C-IV*
0.5, 1, 2 mg (PO)

Buspar® (buspirone)
5, 10, 15, 30 mg (PO)

Insomnia
Rozerem® (ramelteon)
8 mg (PO)

Restoril® (temazepam) *C-IV*
7.5, 15, 22.5, 30 mg (PO)

Lunesta® (eszopiclone) *C-IV* - 1, 2, 3 mg (PO)

Ambien® (zolpidem) *C-IV*
5, 10 mg (PO)
Note: Ambien® CR is an extended-release tablet available in 6.25 and 12.5 mg strengths.

Muscle Spasms
Zanaflex® (tizanidine)
2, 4, 6 mg (PO)

Flexeril® (cyclobenzaprine)
5, 10 mg (PO)

Skelaxin® (metaxalone)
400, 800 mg (PO)

Soma® (carisoprodol) *C-IV*
250, 350 mg (PO)

Robaxin® (methocarbamol)
500, 750 mg (PO)
100 mg/mL (injection solution)
Liorisal® (baclofen)
10, 20 mg (PO)
0.5 mg/mL, 2 mg/mL solution (intrathecal)

Pain
Vicodin® (hydrocodone/acetaminophen) *C-III*
5/300, 5/500 mg (PO)
Note: Vicodin® HP is available in a 10/660 mg tablet and a 10/300 mg tablet;
Vicodin® ES is available in a 7.5/750 mg tablet and a 7.5/300 mg tablet.

Lortab® (hydrocodone/acetaminophen) *C-III*
5/500, 7.5/500, 10/500 mg (PO)
7.5/500 mg/15mL (oral elixir)

Norco® (hydrocodone/acetaminophen) *C-III*
5/325, 7.5/325, 10/325 mg (PO)

Percocet® (oxycodone/acetaminophen) *C-II*
2.5/325, 5/325, 7.5/325, 10/325, 7.5/500, 10/650 mg (PO)

Oxycontin® (oxycodone (ER)) *C-II*
10(ER), 15(ER), 20(ER), 30(ER), 40(ER), 60(ER), 80(ER) mg (PO)

MS Contin® (morphine) *C-II*
15(ER), 30(ER), 60(ER), 100(ER), 200(ER) mg (PO)

Codeine *Also a cough suppressant* *C-II*
15, 30, 60 mg (PO)
30 mg/5mL (oral solution)

Methadone *C-IV*
5, 10, 40 mg (PO)
1, 2, 10 mg/mL (oral solution)
10 mg/mL (injection solution)

Duragesic® (fentanyl) *C-IV*
12, 25, 50, 75, 100 mcg/hour (transdermal patch)

Endocet® (oxycodone/acetaminophen) *C-IV*
5/325, 7.5/325, 10/325, 7.5/500, 10/650 mg (PO)

Demerol® (meperidine) *C-II*
50, 100 mg (PO)
50 mg/mL, 100 mg/mL (injection solution)

Dilaudid® (hydromorphone) *C-II*
2, 4, 8 mg (PO)
1 mg/mL (oral solution)
1, 2, 4 mg/mL (injection solution)

Ultram® (tramadol)
50, 100(ER), 200(ER), 300(ER) mg (PO)

Ultracet® (tramadol/acetaminophen)
37.5/325 mg (PO)

Xilocaine® (lidocaine)
0.5, 1, 2% (injection solution)
2% (mucous membrane solution)
2% (topical jelly)
4% (topical solution)

Lidoderm® (lidocaine)
5% (ER) (topical patch)

Tylenol® #3 (acetaminophen/codeine) *C-III*
30/300 mg (PO)

Migraines
Fioricet® (butalbital/acetaminophen/caffeine)
325/50/40 mg (PO)

Imitrex® (sumatriptan)
25, 50, 100 mg (PO)
6 mg/0.5 mL (SC solution)
5, 20 mg (nasal spray)

Cough
Tussionex® (hydrocodone/chlorpheniramine) *C-III*
8/10 mg/5mL (ER) (oral suspension)

Hycodan® (hydrocodone/homatropine) *C-III*
5/1.5 mg (PO)
Note: Hydromet® is hydrocodone/homatropine 5/1.5 mg/5mL oral syrup.

Tessalon® (benzonatate)
100, 200 mg (PO)

Cheratussin® AC (guaifenesin/codeine) *C-V*
100/10 mg/5mL (oral syrup)

Cheratussin® DAC (guaifenesin/codeine/pseudoephedrine) *C-V*
100/10/30 mg/5mL (oral syrup)

Psychiatric Disorders

Depakote® (divalproex)
125, 250, 500(DR) mg (PO)
Note: Depakote® ER is an extended release tablet available in 250 and 500 mg; Depakote® Sprinkles are capsules whose contents can be sprinkled into soft food and are available in 125 mg capsules.

Seroquel® (quetiapine)
25, 50, 100, 200, 300, 400 mg (PO)
Note: Seroquel® XR is an extended release version of quetiapine available in 50, 150, 200, 300, and 400 mg formulations.

Risperdal® (risperidone)
0.25, 0.5, 1, 2, 3, 4 mg (PO)
1 mg/mL (oral solution)
Note: Risperdal-M® is an orally disintegrating tablet (ODT) available in 0.5, 1, 2, 3, and 4 mg formulations.

Zyprexa® (olanzapine)
2.5, 5, 7.5, 10, 15, 20 mg (PO)
Note: Zyprexa is also available as Zyprexa® Zydis (ODT) and Zyprexa® Relprevv (IM injection).

Geodon® (ziprasidone)
20, 40, 60, 80 mg (PO)
Note: also available as an IM injection.

Haldol® (haloperidol)
0.5, 1, 2, 5, 10, 20 mg (PO)
Note: Haloperidol is also available in an injectable form.

Lithobid®, Eskalith®, Carbolith® (lithium carbonate)
150, 300, 300(ER), 450(CR), 600 mg (PO)

Abilify® (aripiprazole)
2, 5, 10, 15, 20, 30 mg (PO)
1 mg/mL (oral solution)
Note: aripiprazole is also available in a 10 and 15 mg ODT formulation called Abilify® Discmelts and an IM injection known as Abilify® Maintena.

Seizure Disorders

Dilantin® (phenytoin)
50 mg (chewable tablets)
30, 100(ER) mg (PO)
125 mg/5mL (oral suspension)

Tegretol® (carbamazepine)
100 mg (chewable tablets)
200 mg (PO)
100 mg/5mL (oral suspension)

Keppra® (levetiracetam)
250, 500, 750, 1,000 mg (PO)
100 mg/mL (oral solution and IV solution)

Trileptal® (Oxcarbazepine)
150, 300, 600 mg (PO)
300 mg/5mL (oral suspension)

Topamax® (topiramate)
15, 25, 50, 100, 200 mg (PO)

Lamictal® (lamotrigine)
25, 100, 150, 200 mg (PO)
Note: lamotrigine is also available as Lamictal® XR in 25, 50, 100, 200, 250, and 300 extended release tablets.

Neurontin® (gabapentin) *also used for nerve pain*
100, 300, 400, 600, 800 mg (PO)
50 mg/mL (oral solution)

Valium® (diazepam) *also used for anxiety and muscle spasms*
2, 5, 10 mg (PO)
1 mg/mL, 5 mg/mL (oral solution)

Lyrica® (pregabalin) *also used for fibromyalgia/nerve pain* *C-V*
25, 50, 75, 100, 150, 200, 225, 300 mg (PO)
20 mg/mL (oral solution)

Parkinson's Disease
Requip® (ropinirole) *also used to treat restless leg syndrome (RLS)*
0.25, 0.5, 1, 2, 3, 4, 5 mg (PO)
Note: ropinirole is also available as Requip® XL in 2, 4, 6, 8, and 10 mg extended release tablets.

Alzheimer's Disease
Aricept® (donepezil)
5, 5 (ODT), 10, 10(ODT), 23 mg (PO)

Namenda® (memantine)
5, 10 mg (PO)
7(ER), 14(ER), 21(ER), 28(ER) mg (PO)
2 mg/mL (oral solution)

Birth Control
Ortho Evra® (norelgestromin/ethinyl estradiol)
6/0.75 mg (transdermal patch)

Depo-Provera® (medroxyprogesterone)
150 mg/mL, 400 mg/mL (injection suspension)

Menopause Symptoms (Hormone Replacement Therapy)
Premarin® (conjugated estrogens)
0.3, 0.45, 0.625, 0.9, 1.25, 2.5 mg (PO)
0.625 mg/gram (vaginal cream)

Estrace® (estradiol)
0.5, 1, 2 mg (PO)
0.1 mg/gram (vaginal cream)

Evamist® (estradiol)
1.53 mg/actuation (topical spray)

Vagifem® (estradiol)
10 mcg (vaginal tablet)

Overactive Bladder (Urinary Incontinence)
Detrol® (tolterodine)
1, 2 mg (PO)
Note: tolterodine is also available as Detrol® LA in 2 and 4 mg extended release tablets.

Ditropan® (oxybutynin)
5, 5(ER), 10(ER), 15(ER) mg (PO)
1 mg/mL (oral syrup)

Vesicare® (solifenacin)
5, 10 mg (PO)

Nausea/Vomiting (Emesis)
Zofran® (ondansetron)
4, 4(ODT), 8, 8(ODT), 24 mg (PO)
4 mg/5mL (oral solution)
2 mg/mL (injection solution)

Phenergan® (promethazine)
12.5, 25, 50 mg (PO and rectal suppositories)
25 mg/mL, 50 mg/mL (injection solution)

Compazine® (prochlorperazine)
5, 10 mg (PO)

Antivert® (meclizine)
12.5, 25, 50 mg (PO)

Arthritis
Trexall® (methotrexate) MTX *also used to treat some cancers*
5, 7.5, 10, 15 mg (PO)

Inflammation (Steroids)
Medrol® (methylprednisolone)
2, 4, 8, 16, 32 mg (PO)

Deltasone® (prednisone)
1, 2.5, 5, 10, 20, 50 mg (PO)
1 mg/mL, 5 mg/mL (oral solution)

Decadron® (dexamethasone)
0.5, 0.75, 1, 1.5, 2, 4, 6 mg (PO)
0.5 mg/5mL, 5 mg/5mL oral solution
0.5 mg/5mL (elixir)

Cortizone-10® topical (hydrocortisone)
1% (cream, ointment, lotion, gel)

Kenalog® topical (triamcinolone)
0.025, 0.1, 0.5% (cream, ointment, lotion)

Nasacort® AQ (triamcinolone)
55 mcg/actuation (nasal spray)

Inflammation (Non-Steroidal Anti-Inflammatory Drugs (NSAIDs))
Naprosyn® (naproxen)
250, 375, 500 mg (PO)
25 mg/mL (oral suspension)

Motrin®, Advil® (ibuprofen)
100 mg (chewable tablets)
200, 400, 600, 800 mg (PO)
100 mg/5mL oral suspension and IV solution)

Lodine® (etodolac)
200, 300, 400, 400(ER), 500, 500(ER), 600(ER) mg (PO)

Relafen® (nabumetone)
500, 750 mg (PO)

Toradol® (ketorolac)
10 mg (PO)
15 mg/mL, 30 mg/mL (injection solution)

Indocin® (indomethacin) *commonly used in treatment of gout flares*
25, 50, 75(ER) mg (PO)
25 mg/5mL (oral suspension)
50 mg (rectal suppository)

Celebrex® (celecoxib)
50, 100, 200, 400 mg (PO)

Voltaren® (diclofenac)
25, 50, 75, 100(ER) mg (PO)
1% (topical gel)
0.1% (ophthalmic solution)

Mobic® (meloxicam)
7.5, 15 mg (PO)
7.5 mg/5mL (oral suspension)

Allergies
Benadryl® (diphenhydramine)
25, 50 mg (PO)
50 mg/mL (injection solution)
2% (topical gel)
12.5 mg/5mL (oral syrup and oral solution)
12.5 mg (ODT)

Zyrtec® (cetirizine)
5, 10 mg (PO and chewable tablets)
1 mg/mL (oral syrup)
0.025% (ophthalmic solution)

Atarax® (hydroxyzine)
10, 25, 50 mg (PO)
10 mg/5mL (oral syrup)
25 mg/mL, 50 mg/mL (IM solution)

Allegra® (fexofenadine)
30, 30(ODT), 60, 180 mg (PO)
30 mg/5mL (oral suspension)

Flonase® (fluticasone)
50 mcg/actuation (nasal spray)

Claritin® (loratadine)
5 mg (chewable tablets), 5(ODT), 10, 10(ODT) mg (PO)
5 mg/5mL (oral syrup and oral solution)

Nasonex® (mometasone)
50 mcg/actuation (nasal spray)

Gastroesophageal Reflux Disease (GERD)
Prilosec® (omeprazole)
10(DR), 20(DR), 40(DR) mg (PO)

Nexium® (esomeprazole)
20(DR), 40(DR) mg (PO)
2.5, 5, 10, 20, 40 mg/packet (oral packets)
20, 40 mg (powder for IV solution)

Protonix® (pantoprazole)
20, 40 mg (PO)
40 mg/packet (oral packets)
40 mg (powder for IV solution)

Prevacid® (lansoprazole)
15(DR), 15(ODT), 30(DR), 30(ODT) mg (PO)
3 mg/mL (powder for oral suspension)

Dexilant® (dexlansoprazole)
30(DR), 60(DR) mg (PO)

Aciphex® (rabeprazole)
20 mg (PO)

Pepcid® (famotidine)
10, 20, 20 (chewable tablets), 40 mg (PO)
40 mg/5 mL (powder for oral suspension)
0.4 mg/mL, 10 mg/mL (IV solution)

Zantac® (ranitidine)
75, 150, 300 mg (PO)
15 mg/mL (oral syrup)
25 mg/mL (injection solution)

Reglan® (metoclopramide)
5, 10 mg (PO)
5, 10 mg (ODT)
5 mg/5mL (oral syrup and oral solution)
5 mg/mL (IV solution)

Diabetes Mellitus
Byetta® (exenatide) **KEEP REFRIDGERATED**
250 mcg/mL (subcutaneous solution)

Avandia® (rosiglitazone)
2, 4, 8 mg (PO)

Actos® (pioglitazone)
15, 30, 45 mg (PO)

Humulin R®, Novolin R® (regular human insulin) **KEEP REFRIDGERATED**
100 units/mL, 500 units/mL (injection solution)

Lantus® (insulin glargine) **KEEP REFRIDGERATED**
100 units/mL (injection solution)

Glucophage® (metformin)
500, 850, 1,000 mg (PO)
Note: metformin is also available under different brand names in a 500, 750, and
1,000 mg extended-release tablet.

Depression
Wellbutrin® (bupropion)
75, 100 mg (PO)
Note: bupropion is also available in 100, 150, and 200 mg sustained release tablets
(Wellbutrin® SR) and 150 and 300 mg extended release tablets (Wellbutrin® XL).

Remeron® (mirtazapine)
15, 30, 45 mg (PO and ODT)

Prozac® (fluoxetine)
10, 20, 40 mg (PO)
20 mg/5mL (oral syrup and oral solution)
Note: fluoxetine is also available in a 90 mg dose called Prozac® Weekly.

Effexor® (venlafaxine)
25, 37.5, 50, 75, 100 mg (PO)
Note: venlafaxine is also available in 37.5, 75, and 150 mg extended release capsules
(Effexor® XR).

Zoloft® (sertraline)
25, 50, 100 mg (PO)
20 mg/mL (oral solution)

Paxil® (paroxetine)
10, 20, 30, 40 mg (PO)
10 mg/5mL (oral suspension)
Note: paroxetine is also available in 12.5, 25, and 37.5 mg extended release tablets
(Paxil® CR).

Lexapro® (escitalopram)
5, 10, 20 mg (PO)
5 mg/5mL (oral solution)

Celexa® (citalopram)
10, 20, 40 mg (PO)
10 mg/5mL (oral solution)

Cymbalta® (duloxetine)
20(DR), 30(DR), 60(DR) mg (PO)

Desyrel® (trazodone) *also used to treat insomnia*
50, 100 mg (PO)
Note: trazodone is also available in 150 mg and 300 mg extended release tablets.

Elavil® (amitriptyline)
10, 25, 50, 75, 100, 150 mg (PO)

Asthma
AccuNeb® (albuterol inhalation solution)
0.021%, 0.042%, 0.083% (inhalation solution)

Proventil®, ProAir®, Ventolin® (albuterol inhaler)
0.09 mg/actuation (inhaler)

Singulair® (montelukast)
4, 5 mg (chewable tablet)
10 mg (PO)
4 mg (oral packet)

Advair® (fluticasone/salmeterol)
100/50, 250/50, 500/50 mcg (inhalation disk)
45/21, 115/21, 230/21 mcg/actuation (inhaler)

COPD
Atrovent® (ipratropium inhalation solution)
0.02% (inhalation solution)
0.017 mg/actuation (inhaler)
0.03%, 0.05% (nasal spray)

Spiriva® (tiotropium capsules for inhalation)
18 mcg (inhalation capsule)

Cardiac Arrhythmias
Lanoxin® (digoxin)
0.125, 0.25 mg (PO)
0.25 mg/mL (IV solution)

Pacerone® (amiodarone)
100, 200, 400 mg (PO)

Blood Clot Treatment/Prevention
Heparin
10, 100, 1000, 2500, 5000, 10000, 20000 units/mL (injection solution)

Coumadin®, Jantoven® (warfarin)
1, 2, 2.5, 3, 4, 5, 6, 7.5, 10 mg (PO)
5 mg (powder for IV solution)

Ecotrin® (aspirin) *also used for pain and fever*
81, 325, 500 mg (PO)

Plavix® (clopidogrel)
75, 300 mg (PO)

Lovenox® (enoxaparin)
30 mg/0.3mL, 40 mg/0.4mL, 60 mg/0.6mL, 80 mg/0.8mL, 100 mg/mL, 120 mg/0.8mL, 150 mg/mL (subcutaneous solution)

Angina/Heart Attack Prevention (Vasodilators)
Apresoline® (hydralazine)
10, 25, 50, 100 mg (PO)
20 mg/mL (injection solution)

Imdur® (isosorbide mononitrate)
10, 20, 30(ER), 60(ER), 120(ER) mg (PO)

Nitro-bid® transdermal ointment (nitroglycerin)
2% (transdermal ointment)

Nitro-dur® transdermal patch (nitroglycerin)
0.1, 0.2, 0.3, 0.4, 0.6, 0.8 mg/hr (transdermal patch)

Nitrostat® sublingual (nitroglycerin)
0.3, 0.4, 0.6 mg (sublingual tablet)

Hypertension (High Blood Pressure)
Dyrenium® (triamterene)
50, 100 mg (PO)

Maxzide®, Dyazide® (hydrochlorthiazide/triamterene)
25/37.5, 25/50, 50/75 mg (PO)

Norvasc® (amlodipine)
2.5, 5, 10 mg (PO)

Atacand® (candesartan)
4, 8, 16, 32 mg (PO)

Accupril® (quinapril)
5, 10, 20, 40 mg (PO)

Avalide® (irbesartan/hydrochlorothiazide)
12.5/150, 12.5/300, 25/300 mg (PO)

Hyzaar® (losartan/hydrochlorothiazide)
12.5/50, 12.5/100, 25/100 mg (PO)

Inderal® (propranolol) *also commonly used for migraines*
10, 20, 40, 60, 80 mg (PO)
Note: propranolol is also available as 60, 80, 120, and 160 mg extended release
capsules (Inderal® LA, Innopran® XL).

Avapro® (irbesartan)
75, 150, 300 mg (PO)

Cozaar® (losaratan)
25, 50, 100 mg (PO)

Microzide® (hydrochlorothiazide)
12.5, 25, 50 mg (PO)

Cardizem®, Tiazac® (diltiazem) *also used for cardiac arrhythmias*
30, 60, 60(ER), 90, 90(ER), 120, 120(ER), 180(ER), 240(ER), 300(ER), 360(ER), 420(ER)
mg (PO)
5 mg/mL (IV solution)

Isoptin®, Calan® (verapamil) *also used for cardiac arrhythmias*
40, 80, 100(ER), 120, 120(ER), 180(ER), 200(ER), 240(ER), 300(ER), 360(ER) mg (PO)
2.5 mg/mL (IV solution)

Vasotec® (enalapril)
2.5, 5, 10, 20 mg (PO)

Benicar® (olmesartan)
5, 20, 40 mg (PO)

Catapress® (clonidine)
0.1, 0.2, 0.3 mg (PO)
0.1, 0.2, 0.3 mg/24-hr (transdermal patch)

Altace® (ramipril)
1.25, 2.5, 5, 10 mg (PO)

Coreg® (carvedilol)
3.125, 6.25, 12.5, 25 mg (PO)
Note: carvedilol is also available in 10, 20, 40, and 80 mg extended release capsules (Coreg® CR).

Lasix® (furosemide) *also used to treat edema*
20, 40, 80 mg (PO)
10 mg/mL (injection solution)

Aldactone® (spironolactone)
25, 50, 100 mg (PO)

Nifediac®, Procardia® (nifedipine)
10, 20, 30(ER), 60(ER), 90(ER) mg (PO)

Diovan® (valsartan)
40, 80, 160, 320 mg (PO)

Prinivil®, Zestril® (lisinopril)
2.5, 5, 10, 20, 30, 40 mg (PO)

Lotrel® (amlodipine/benazepril)
2.5/10, 5/10, 5/20, 5/40, 10/20, 10/40 mg (PO)

Norvasc® (amlodipine)
2.5, 5, 10 mg (PO)

Lopressor® (metoprolol tartrate (IR)) *also used for cardiac arrhythmias*
50, 100 mg (PO)
1 mg/mL (injection solution)

Toprol® XL (metoprolol succinate (ER)) *also used for cardiac arrhythmias*
25, 50, 100, 200 mg (PO)

Tenormin® (atenolol)
25, 50, 100 mg (PO)

High Cholesterol
Niaspan® (niacin)
500 mg, 750 mg, 1,000 mg ER (PO)

Zocor® (simvastatin)
5, 10, 20, 40, 80 mg (PO)

Mevacor® (lovastatin)
10, 20, 40 mg (PO)

Crestor® (rosuvastatin)
5, 10, 20, 40 mg (PO)

Tricor® (fenofibrate)
48, 145 mg (PO)

Pravachol® (pravastatin)
10, 20, 40, 80 mg (PO)

Lipitor® (atorvastatin)
10, 20, 40, 80 mg (PO)

Vytorin® (ezetemibe/simvastatin)
10/10, 10/20, 10/40, 10/80 mg (PO)

Zetia® (ezetimibe)
10 mg (PO)

Cardiac Arrest
AtroPen® (atropine)
various concentrations (SC, IM, IV)

Gout
Zyloprim® (allopurinol)
100, 300 mg (PO)
various concentrations (IV)

Colcrys® (colchicine)
 0.6 mg (PO)

Prostate Cancer
Lupron® (luprolide)
various concentrations (SC, IV)

Fungal Infections
Nystop® (nystatin)
100,000 units/gram (topical powder)
Note: nystatin is also available in a 100,000 unit/mL oral suspension.

Diflucan® (fluconazole)
50, 100, 150, 200 mg (PO)
10 mg/mL and 40 mg/mL (oral suspension)
2 mg/mL (IV)

Viral Infections
Tamiflu® (oseltamivir)
75 mg (PO)
6 mg/mL (oral suspension)

Valtrex® (valacyclovir)
500 mg, 1 gram (PO)

Zovirax® (acyclovir)
200, 400, 800 mg (PO)
200mg/5mL (oral suspension)
5% (topical cream and topical ointment)

Bacterial Infections
Vancocin® (vancomycin)
125 mg, 250 mg (PO)
various concentrations (IV)

Ery-tab® (erythromycin)
250, 333, 500(DR) mg (PO)

Avelox® (moxifloxacin)
400 mg (PO)
various concentrations (IV)

Penicillin (Generic Only)
250, 500 mg (PO)
125 mg/5mL, 250 mg/5mL (oral suspension)
various concentrations (IV)

Tetracycline (Generic Only)
250, 500 mg (PO)

Falgyl® (metronidazole)
250, 375, 500, 750 mg ER (PO)
various concentrations (IV)

Omnicef® (cefdinir)
300 mg (PO)
125 mg/5mL, 250 mg/5mL (oral suspension)

Vibramycin® (doxycycline)
100 mg (PO)
25 mg/5mL, 50 mg/5mL (oral suspension)

Augmentin® (amoxicillin/clavulanate)
250/125, 500/125, 875/125, 1,000/62.5 mg ER (PO)
125/31.25 mg/5mL, 250/62.5 mg/5mL (oral suspension)

Keflex® (cephalexin)
250, 500, 750 mg (PO)
125 mg/5mL, 250 mg/5mL (oral suspension)

Bactrim®, Septra® (sulfamethoxazole/trimethoprim)
80/400 mg, 160/800 mg (PO)
400/200 mg/5mL (oral suspension)

Cipro® (ciprofloxacin)
100, 250, 500, 750 mg (PO)
250 mg/5 mL, 500 mg/5 mL (oral suspension)
10 mg/mL (IV solution)

Cleocin® (clindamycin)
75, 150, 300 mg (PO)
6 mg/mL, 12 mg/mL, 18 mg/mL, 150 mg/mL (IV solution)
1% (Topical Gel, Jelly, Lotion, Pad, Solution, and Foam)
2% (vaginal cream)
100 mg (vaginal suppository)

Amoxil® (amoxicillin)
125, 200, 250, 400, 500, 775 ER, 875 mg (PO)
125 mg/5mL, 200 mg/5mL, 250 mg/5mL, 400 mg/5mL (oral suspension)

Z-pak® (azithromycin)
250 mg (PO)

Zithromax® (azithromycin)
250, 500, 600 mg (PO)
1 gram packet, 100 mg/5mL, 200 mg/5mL (oral suspension)
500 mg (powder for IV solution)
Note: AzaSite® is azithromycin 1% ophthalmic solution.

Levaquin® (levofloxacin)
250, 500, 750 mg (PO)
25 mg/mL (oral solution)
5 mg/mL (IV solution)

Biaxin® (clarithromycin)
250, 500 mg (PO)
125 mg/5mL, 250 mg/5mL (oral suspension)
Note: Biaxin® XL is a 500 mg extended-release tablet.

Attention Deficit Hyperactivity Disorder (ADHD)
Ritalin® (methylphenidate)
5, 10, 20 mg (PO)
Note: Ritalin® LA is an extended-release capsule available in 10, 20, 30, and 40 mg strengths.

Concerta® (methylphenidate (ER))
18 (ER), 27 (ER), 36 (ER), 54 (ER) mg (PO)

Adderall® (amphetamine/dextroamphetamine salts)
5, 7.5, 10, 12.5, 15, 20, 30 mg (PO)
Note: Adderall® XR is an extended-release capsule available in 5, 10, 15, 20, 25, and 30 mg strengths.

Strattera® (atomoxetine)
10, 18, 25, 40, 60, 80, 100 mg (PO)

Provigil® (modafinil) *also used to treat daytime sleepiness*
100, 200 mg (PO)

Erectile Dysfunction (ED)
Viagra® (sildenafil)
25, 50, 100 mg (PO)
Note: Revatio® (sildenafil) is used for treatment of pulmonary hypertension and is available in a 20 mg tablet and a 10 mg/12.5mL IV solution.

Levitra® (vardenafil)
2.5, 5, 10, 20 (PO)
Note: Staxyn® (vardenafil) is available in a 10 mg orally disintegrating tablet (ODT).

Cialis® (tadalafil)
2.5, 5, 10, 20 (PO)

Benign Prostatic Hyperplasia (BPH)
Flomax® (tamsulosin)
0.4 mg (PO)

Hytrin® (terazosin)
2, 5, 10 mg (PO)

Irregular Menstrual Bleeding
Provera® (medroxyprogesterone)
2.5, 5, 10 mg (PO)

In this section we cover the pharmacology of some popular drug classes including uses (Indications), mechanisms of action (MoA), side effects (SE), and common drug interactions (DI). Focus on the highlighted details.

ANGIOTENSIN CONVERTING ENZYME (ACE) INHIBITORS

Examples: Prinivil®/Zestril® (lisinopril), Vasotec® (enalapril), Lotensin® (benazepril)

Indications: Hypertension, Heart Failure, Myocardial Infarction (heart attack), Renal Protection in Diabetes Mellitus

MoA: Inhibits angiotensin converting enzyme (ACE), thus preventing the conversion of angiotensin I to angiotensin II. Angiotensin II is a potent vasoconstrictor (constricts blood vessels leading to increased blood pressure). Angiotensin II also stimulates secretion of aldosterone, a mineralocorticoid secreted from the kidneys, which increases sodium levels in the blood. Since water follows sodium, aldosterone secretion ultimately leads to an increase in blood volume and an increase in blood pressure.

SE: Dry cough, hypotension, hyperkalemia, anaphylaxis (rare).

DI: Potassium supplements used together with ACE inhibitors may lead to dangerously high potassium levels in the blood → cardiac arrhythmias.

Notes: Fetal toxicity (Pregnancy category X). About 20% of patients on ACE inhibitors experience a dry, nonproductive cough. The only way to eliminate this side effect is to discontinue the ACE inhibitor. Switch to an ARB for the same pharmacologic effect without the dry cough side effect.

Examples: Cozaar® (losartan), Avapro® (irbesartan), Diovan® (valsartan), Benicar® (olmesartan), Micardis® (telmisartan)

Indications: Hypertension, Heart Failure, Myocardial Infarction (heart attack) Stroke Prevention, Renal Protection in Diabetes Mellitus

MoA: Antagonizes angiotensin II at type 1 angiotensin II receptors (AT1 receptors) found on the blood vessels and heart. The antagonism of angiotensin II leads to relaxation of vascular smooth muscle.

SE: Fatigue, dizziness, hyperkalemia, hypotension, angioedema (rare), anaphylaxis (rare). Since the ARBs do not interfere with bradykinin metabolism, they are not associated with the dry cough side effect seen with ACE inhibitors.

DI: Since ARBs can increase potassium levels, potassium supplements and salt substitutes can increase the risk of hyperkalemia.

Notes: Fetal/neonatal toxicity (Pregnancy category X).

Examples: Microzide® (hydrochlorothiazide), Diuril® (chlorthiazide), Zaroxolyn® (metolazone)

Indications: Hypertension, Peripheral Edema

MoA: Decreases NaCl reabsorption at the distal convoluted tubule (DTC) of the nephron by inhibiting the Na+–Cl- symporter. As a result, more sodium remains in the urine. Water follows sodium, thus urine output increases (causing blood volume to decrease).

SE: Hyperglycemia, Hyperuricemia, Hypokalemia, Muscle Cramps (related to electrolyte imbalances), Cardiac Arrhythmias (also related to electrolyte imbalances), Photosensitivity (predisposition to sunburn), Stevens-Johnson Syndrome (SJS; rare).

DI: Additive hypotension when combined with other drugs that can cause hypotension; Additive hypokalemia when administered with loop diuretics; Works against drugs like allopurinol which work to lower uric acid levels; Can increase blood sugar (monitor blood sugar more closely in diabetics starting or stopping thiazides).

Notes: Thiazides contain a sulfonamide group, which may cause an allergic reaction in patients with a sulfa allergy. Unlike loop diuretics, thiazides have a ceiling effect on diuresis (can only increase urine output up to a certain extent). Judging from the image below, one might venture to guess that diuretics cause hyperkalemia; however, further down stream in the nephron, the body tries to compensate for the excess sodium in the urine by making a last-ditch effort to exchange it for potassium. In this effort, the body loses a lot of potassium and we end up seeing hypokalemia.

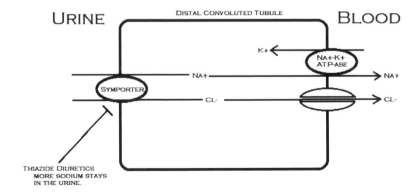

```
********************************************************************************
```

**Drug Interaction –
The "Triple Whammy"**

The "Triple Whammy" is the term for the drug interaction between three medications – an NSAID, an ACE or ARB, and a diuretic. When used together, these three medications can cause acute renal damage. NSAIDs inhibit production of prostaglandins, chemicals that work to keep blood vessels feeding the kidneys dilated. ACEs and ARBs cause vasodilation of the efferent arteriole, reducing glomerular filtration pressure. Diuretics cause a reduction in blood flow to the kidneys by reducing blood volume. In other words, all three of these drugs work in different ways that ultimately reduces blood flow to the kidneys. When blood supply is diminished, the cells starve and the organ fails.

```
********************************************************************************
```

POTASSIUM-SPARING DIURETICS

Examples: Dyrenium® (triamterene), Midamor® (amiloride), Inspra® (eplerenone), Aldactone® (spironolactone)

Indications: Hypertension, Heart Failure, Lithium-induced Polyuria

MoA: Triamterene and Amiloride block sodium-potassium exchange, leading to increased urinary sodium and decreased urinary potassium. Eplerenone and Spironolactone are steroidal compounds that work by antagonizing aldosterone receptors. Aldosterone is a potent mineralocorticoid (causes sodium and water retention).

SE: Spironolactone has some hormonal side effects due to its steroidal chemical structure which can cause gynecomastia in males and breast tenderness in females.

DI: Use of potassium supplements and salt substitutes increases the risk of hyperkalemia.

Notes: Drugs from this class are poor diuretics compared to loops and thiazides. Potassium-sparing diuretics can be used in conjunction with loops or thiazides to help avoid potassium imbalances.

Examples: Bumex® (bumetanide), Demadex® (torsemide), Lasix® (furosemide)

Indications: Hypertension, Edema

MoA: Loop diuretics work by blocking the Na-K-Cl2 symporter (a protein that functions to transport sodium, potassium, and chloride ions in a 1:1:2 ratio from the urine to the blood) in the thick ascending limb of the Loop of Henle (part of the nephron). Since water follows sodium, this results in increased urine output to decrease blood volume (decreases blood pressure/edema).

SE: (Virtually the same side effects as seen with the thiazide diuretics) Hyperglycemia, Hyperuricemia, Hypokalemia, Muscle Cramps (related to electrolyte imbalances), Cardiac Arrhythmias (also related to electrolyte imbalances), Photosensitivity (predisposition to sunburn), SJS (rare).

DI: (Virtually the same drug interactions as seen with the thiazide diuretics) Additive hypotension when combined with other drugs that can cause hypotension; Additive hypokalemia when administered with loop diuretics; Works against drugs like allopurinol which work to lower uric acid levels; Can increase blood sugar (monitor blood sugar more closely in diabetics starting or stopping thiazides).

Notes: Loop diuretics are the most effective diuretics available. Unlike the thiazides, loop diuretics have no ceiling effect on diuresis. Loop diuretics have the potential to cause life-threatening fluid and electrolyte depletion if used improperly.

****
Pneumonic for Loop Diuretics:

"Beau-Ti-Ful"

When you break the word "beautiful" down into its three syllables (beau- -ti- -ful), you see that each syllable begins with a letter corresponding to the first letter of the generic name of a loop diuretic.
The "**B**" in **Beau**- corresponds to the "**B**" in **Bumetanide**.
The "**T**" in -**Ti**- corresponds to the "**T**" in **Torsemide**.
The "**F**" in –**Ful** corresponds to the "**F**" in **Furosemide**.
****

Examples: Flomax® (tamsulosin), Hytrin® (terazosin), Cardura® (doxazosin), Minipress® (prazosin), Uroxatral® (afluzosin), Rapaflo® (silodosin)

Indications: Benign Prostatic Hyperplasia (BPH), Hypertension

MoA: Alpha₁ blockers prevent stimulation of alpha₁ receptors. There are three subtypes of alpha₁ receptors. Stimulation of the alpha$_{1A}$ receptor subtype causes contraction of smooth muscles in the bladder neck and prostate. Benign prostatic hyperplasia is characterized by an enlarged prostate that obstructs urine outflow at the level of the bladder neck (the prostate gland encompasses the bladder neck). By selectively blocking the alpha$_{1A}$ receptor subtype, smooth muscle tissue in the prostate and bladder neck are relaxed, allowing for unobstructed urine outflow. Non-selective alpha₁ blockers (not targeted specifically at alpha$_{1A}$) cause relaxation of smooth muscle tissue that lines the blood vessels all through the body, resulting in decreased peripheral vascular resistance and blood pressure.

SE: Orthostatic hypotension (blood pressure drops dramatically upon standing), dizziness, syncope, priapism.

DI: Increased risk of hypotension when used with other drugs that lower blood pressure.

Examples: Catapress®/Kapvay® (clonidine), Intuniv®/Tenex® (guanfacine), Aldomet® (methyldopa)

Indications: Hypertension, ADHD

MoA: Activates aplha₂-adrenergic receptors. Alpha₂-adrenergic receptors are "autoreceptors." They are found on sympathetic nerve terminals (nerves that release norepinephrine). When activated, alpha₂ receptors provide negative feedback to the nerve terminal, which results in decreased norepinephrine output. In simplified terms, activation of alpha2-adrenergic receptors by drugs like clonidine, guanfacine, and methyldopa leads to reduced norepinephrine output by the nervous system. Less norepinephrine causes lower blood pressure.

SE: Bradycardia (slow heart rate), rebound hypertension (upon withdrawal), dry mouth, impotence, fatigue.

DI: Increased risk of hypotension when used with other drugs that decrease blood pressure. Also increases risk of bradycardia when used with drugs that decrease heart rate (e.g. diltiazem, verapamil, and beta-blockers).

Examples: Toprol XL®/Lopressor® (metoprolol), Tenormin® (atenolol), Coreg® (carvedilol), Inderal® (propranolol)

Indications: Hypertension, Angina, Atrial Fibrillation, Myocardial Infarction, Migraines

MoA: β-blockers antagonize beta-adrenergic receptors, preventing catecholamines (dopamine, norepinephrine, epinephrine) from binding. This results in decreased chronotropy (slower heart rate), decreased inotropy (less forceful heart beats), and vasodilation (decreased blood pressure).

SE: Bradycardia, hypotension, dizziness, fatigue, constipation, diarrhea, dry eyes, male impotence.

DI: NSAIDs decrease production of renal prostaglandins, leading to an increase in blood pressure. Some β-blockers interfere with the elimination of diazepam, resulting in higher than expected blood concentrations of diazepam (note: atenolol does not interfere with diazepam metabolism).

Notes: β-blockers should be taken with food. This slows the rate of absorption, decreasing the potential for side effects. Also note that β-blockers blunt the sympathetic response to hypoglycemia, which typically includes sweating, palpitations, and tremor. For diabetic patients on β-blockers, sweating is the only sign of hypoglycemia that remains. Symptoms of more severe cases of hypoglycemia may involve seizure or coma. Abrupt cessation may cause exacerbations of angina, potentially leading to myocardial infarction. When discontinuing, the dose should be decreased gradually over one to two weeks.

Examples: Norvasc® (amlodipine), Procardia® (nifedipine), Cardizem® (diltiazem), Isoptin® (verapamil)

Indications: Hypertension, Angina, Coronary Artery Disease

MoA: Calcium channel blockers work by reducing the flow of calcium ion into cardiac and vascular smooth muscle cells, which rely on calcium for contraction. Resultantly, you see relaxation of vascular smooth muscle (thus a reduction in peripheral blood vessels → treats high blood pressure) and a reduction in cardiac contractility (the heart contracts less forcefully, thus the heart demands less oxygen → treats angina*).

SE: Fatigue, edema.

DI: Patients on amlodipine should not take more than 20 mg of simvastatin daily due to increased risk of rhabdomyolysis; strong inhibitors of CYP3A4 increase plasma concentrations of amlodipine, which could lead to hypotension and an increase in side effects. The risk of hypotension increases when taken with other drugs that lower blood pressure.

Notes: *Angina is essentially chest pain that results from inadequate blood flow to the heart (blood functions to supply cells with oxygen, so inadequate blood flow means inadequate oxygen supply).

Examples: Viagra®/Revatio® (sildenafil), Cialis® (tadalafil), Levitra® (vardenafil)

Indications: Erectile Dysfunction, Pulmonary Arterial Hypertension (Revatio® only)

MoA: PDE-5 inhibitors inhibit the enzyme phosphodiesterase-5. Inhibition of PDE-5 prolongs the effect of nitric oxide (a potent vasodilator → increases blood flow). Phosphodiesterase-5 is an enzyme mainly present in pulmonary vascular smooth muscle (i.e. the blood vessels inside the lungs) and the corpus cavernosum (i.e. the tissue that comprises the penis), thus PDE-5 inhibitors work to increase blood flow to these areas.

SE: Hypotension, headache, epistaxis (nosebleed), priapism (a persistent, painful erection)

DI: Increased risk of hypotension when used with other medications that can lower blood pressure (especially nitroglycerin). Increased risk of epistaxis (nosebleed) when used with anticoagulants or antiplatelets.

Examples: Zocor® (simvastatin), Lipitor® (atorvastatin), Crestor® (rosuvastatin), Pravachol® (pravastatin), Lescol® (lovastatin)

Indications: Hypercholesterolemia (high cholesterol)

MoA: Humans obtain cholesterol from two sources: (1) food and (2) the cholesterol the body synthesizes naturally. Statins work by inhibiting the enzyme HMG-CoA reductase, which is a key enzyme involved in the synthesis of cholesterol. Most cholesterol synthesis occurs during the night, so statins are typically more effective when taken at night. Certain statins (e.g. atorvastatin, rosuvastatin) are eliminated from the body at a very slow rate (a long half-life) and for this reason it is not necessary to take them at night - they can be taken at any time of the day. Patients on a statin should also implement dietary changes to reduce cholesterol intake.

SE: Muscle aches, constipation, liver impairment, myopathy, rhabdomyolysis (rare)

DI: Most drug interactions involving statins are ones that lead to an increased risk of myopathy. For drugs in this class, then enzymes responsible for metabolism vary from drug to drug, but in general drugs that inhibit or induce certain CYP450 enzymes (e.g. ketoconazole, cyclosporine, carbamazepine, high quantities of grapefruit juice) lead to decreased or increased metabolism of statins. Enzyme inhibitors can cause decreased metabolism of the statin and the statin builds up in the body, causing more side effects (i.e. myopathy). Enzyme inducers cause increased metabolism of statins, decreasing the effectiveness of the statin.

Notes: Pregnancy Category X.

Anti-arrhythmic Agents

Examples: Pacerone® (amiodarone), Lanoxin® (digoxin), Quinalan® (quinidine), Norpace® (disopyramide), Xylocaine® (lidocaine), Rythmol® (propafenone), Tambocor® (flecainide), Betapace® (sotalol), Tikosyn® (dofetilide)

Indications: Cardiac Arrhythmias

MoA: Antiarrhythmics essentially slow down/stabilize the nerve impulses that travel through the heart tissue.

SE: New or worsened arrhythmias, liver damage, visual disturbances, dizziness, fatigue, nausea/vomiting

DI: When taken with drugs that prolong the QT interval (e.g. citalopram, moxifloxacin, tacrolimus, ziprasidone), life-threatening cardiac arrhythmias can result.

Examples: AtroPen® (atropine), Antivert® (meclizine), Dramamine® (dimenhydrinate), Transderm-Scop® (scopolamine)

Indications: Nausea/Vomiting, Vertigo, Delirium Tremens

MoA: Anticholinergics work by inhibiting the action of acetylcholine (Ach). Acetylcholine is a parasympathetic neurotransmitter. The parasympathetic nervous system is responsible for "rest and digest" activity (e.g. slowing of the heart, contraction of GI smooth muscle, increased digestive gland secretions, constriction of the pupils, and constriction of the bronchioles) whereas the sympathetic nervous system is responsible for "fight or flight" activity (e.g. increased heart rate, dilation of pupils, dilation of bronchioles). Anticholinergic drugs are also known as "parasympatholytics" ("-lytic" coming from the Greek word for breaking) because they oppose the effects of parasympathetic nervous system stimulation.

SE: Cholinergic effects are summarized in the acronym "SLUDGE."

> S – Salivation
> L – Lacrimation
> U – Urination
> D – Defecation
> G – Glandular Secretions
> E – Emesis

Since anticholinergic drugs block, or reduce, cholinergic activity, side effects are predictable (e.g. dry mouth, dry eye, urinary retention, constipation).

DI: Anticholinergics should not be used in patients with narrow angle glaucoma, as they will cause an increase in intraocular pressure (worsening of the glaucoma). Also, aluminum and magnesium-containing antacids may decrease absorption of orally administered anticholinergics.

Examples: Prozac® (fluoxetine), Paxil® (paroxetine), Zoloft® (sertraline), Celexa® (citalopram), Lexapro® (escitalopram), Luvox® (fluvoxamine)

Indications: Depression, Behavioral Disorders, Eating Disorders

MoA: Serotonin (chemical name: 5-hydroxytryptamine (5-HT)) is a neurotransmitter that plays key roles in depression, behavior, eating, and nausea/vomiting. Serotonin must remain available in the open space between neurons (known as the synaptic cleft) to exert an effect. When neurons reabsorb (or "reuptake") serotonin, the serotonin is effectively removed from the synaptic cleft and rendered inactive. SSRIs inhibit the reuptake of serotonin, allowing the neurotransmitter to remain in the synaptic cleft where it has more time to exert its effect.

SE: Weight gain/loss, reduced sex drive, dry mouth, nausea, diarrhea, serotonin syndrome.

****
Symptoms of Serotonin Syndrome
Changes in mental status (e.g. agitation, confusion, hallucinations), pressured speech, tremor*, rigidity, diarrhea, fever, sweating, flushing, and seizures.

*Tremor is the hallmark symptom of serotonin syndrome.
****

DI: Increased risk of bleeding when used with NSAIDs, anticoagulants, and/or antiplatelets. Increased risk of serotonin syndrome when used with other medications that increase the effect of serotonin (e.g. SNRIs, triptans, Ultram® (tramadol)).

Notes: All antidepressants have the potential to cause suicidal ideation and behavior in patients age 24 and under.

Examples: Cymbalta® (duloxetine), Effexor® (venlafaxine), Pristiq® (desvenlafaxine), Savella® (milnacipran)

Indications: Depression, Eating Disorders, Generalized Anxiety Disorder, Diabetic Peripheral Neuropathy

MoA: SNRIs have a mechanism similar to SSRIs, but they also inhibit the reuptake of norepinephrine (also known as noradrenalin).

SE: Side effects of SNRIs are similar to those of SSRIs (e.g. serotonin syndrome), but with additional cardiovascular side effects (e.g. heart palpitations, increased blood pressure, tachycardia). Common side effects include dry mouth, nausea, headache, fatigue, and dizziness.

DI: Increased risk of serotonin syndrome when taken with other drugs that increase the activity of serotonin (e.g. SSRIs, triptans, Ultram® (tramadol)).

Examples: Apidra® (insulin glulisine), NovoLog® (insulin aspart), Humalog® (insulin lispro), Humulin R®/Novolin R® (regular human insulin), Humulin N®/Novolin N® (insulin NPH), Lantus® (insulin glargine), Levemir® (insulin detemir), Tresiba® (insulin degludec)

Indications: Type I Diabetes Mellitus, Type II Diabetes Mellitus

MoA: Insulin stimulates cellular uptake of glucose from the blood. There are several different insulin formulations. They are categorized based on how quickly they start working (onset of action) and how long they work (duration of action).

Category	Brand Name	Onset of Action	Duration of Action
Rapid Acting	Apidra®, Humalog®, NovoLog®	15 - 30 min.	3 - 6 hours
Short Acting	Humulin R®, Novolin R®	30 - 60 min.	6 - 10 hours
Intermediate Acting	Humulin N®, Novolin N®	1 - 2 hours	16 - 24 hours
Long Acting	Lantus®, Levemir®	1 - 2 hours	24 hours
Ultra Long Acting	Tresiba®	1 hour	24 - 40 hours

SE: Hypoglycemia, redness/swelling/itching at injection site

DI: Several drugs (e.g. thyroid hormones, diuretics, corticosteroids) can increase blood sugar, opposing the effect of insulin. Likewise, several drugs (e.g. oral antidiabetics, fibrates) can decrease blood sugar and have additive blood sugar lowering effects.

Notes: **KEEP REFRIDGERATED** until dispensed. Insulin expires 28 days after the rubber stopper of the vial is punctured with a needle. With the exception of U-500 insulin, the stock concentration of all insulin is 100 units per milliliter (each 0.01 mL of liquid contains 1 unit of insulin). With U-500 insulin, the concentration is 500 units per milliliter.

****
Insulin Formulations Available Without a Prescription (OTC)

Novolin N	Novolin R	Novolin 70/30
Humulin N	Humulin R	Humulin 70/30

****

About Diabetes
Cells need to be able to use glucose in order to survive. Insulin gives cells the ability to use glucose. Patients with type I diabetes do not produce enough insulin to survive, therefore these patients require insulin. Patients with type II diabetes do not always require insulin injections. Often times, they can control their blood sugar levels with diet, exercise, and oral antidiabetics (sulfonylureas, DPP-4 inhibitors, metformin, and others).

Examples: Glucophage®, Fortamet® (metformin)

Indications: Type II Diabetes Mellitus

MoA: Lowers blood glucose by three mechanisms:
1. Decreases amount of glucose produced by the liver.
2. Decreases intestinal absorption of glucose.
3. Improves cellular response to insulin.

Note: Metformin does not work by increasing insulin secretion; therefore, it does not have the potential to cause hypoglycemia as some other oral antidiabetics do.

SE: Lactic acidosis, vitamin B12 deficiency, diarrhea, nausea/vomiting

DI: Cimetidine can increase metformin levels by up to 50%.

DIPEPTIDYL PEPTIDASE-4 (DPP-4) INHIBITORS

Examples: Januvia® (sitagliptin), Onglyza® (saxagliptin), Tradjenta® (linagliptin), Nesina® (alogliptin)

Indications: Type II Diabetes Mellitus

MoA: DPP-4 inhibitors lower blood glucose by preventing the degradation of incretins. Incretins are naturally present in the human body. They increase insulin secretion and decrease glucagon secretion. By preserving incretins, more glucose is absorbed by cells via insulin and less glucose is mobilized into the bloodstream by glucagon.

SE: Hypoglycemia (low risk), musculoskeletal pain, headache, upper respiratory infection, Stevens-Johnson Syndrome (SJS; rare).

DI: Increased risk of hypoglycemia when used in combination with sulfonylureas (especially glyburide) and/or insulin. CYP3A4 inducers (e.g. rifampin) can reduce the effect of saxagliptin and linagliptin. CYP3A4 inhibitors (e.g. ketoconazole, clarithromycin) can increase the effect of saxagliptin and linagliptin.

Examples: Amaryl® (glimepiride), Glucotrol® (glipizide), DiaBeta®/Micronase® (glyburide), Tolinase® (tolazamide), Tol-tab® (tolbutamide), Diabinese® (chlorpropamide)

Indications: Type II Diabetes Mellitus

MoA: Cells obtain the fuel they need to survive from glucose in the blood. Insulin allows cells to take up glucose from the blood. In type II diabetes, the cells are insensitive to insulin, not enough insulin is being secreted, or both. Since the glucose is not being used by the cells, it builds up in the blood. The high concentrations of glucose in the blood damage the blood vessels and nerves. Severe damage to the blood vessels of the kidneys (leading to renal failure) and the nerves of the eye (leading to blindness) are typical of diabetes. Sulfonylureas are secretagogues, meaning they stimulate insulin secretion.

SE: Since sulfonylureas stimulate insulin secretion, hypoglycemia is a side effect (more severe with glyburide; especially when dietary intake is limited). Another common side effect is weight gain (also more severe with glyburide).

DI: Many drugs (e.g. quinolones, anticoagulants, azole antifungals, MAOIs) can increase the hypoglycemic effect of sulfonylureas. Likewise, many drugs (e.g. thyroid hormones, diuretics, corticosteroids, beta-blockers, calcium channel blockers) can reduce the effect of sulfonylureas. Also worth noting, alcohol can prolong the effect of glipizide and cause a disulfiram-like reaction in patients taking chlorpropamide.

Notes: Use of 2ND generation sulfonylureas (glimepiride, glipizide, glyburide) is preferred over 1ST generation sulfonylureas (tolazamide, tolbutamide, chlorpropamide).

Examples: Prilosec® (omeprazole), Protonix® (pantoprazole), Prevacid® (lansoprazole), AciPhex® (rabeprazole), Nexium® (esomeprazole)

Indications: Gastroesophageal Reflux Disease (GERD), Peptic Ulcer Disease (PUD), Barrett's Esophagus

MoA: An enzyme known as Hydrogen-Potassium ATPase, or the proton pump, is responsible for secreting acid (i.e. hydrogen ions) into the interior of the stomach by taking ions of potassium out of the stomach and placing hydrogen ions into the stomach. Proton pump inhibitors block this enzyme and prevent it from functioning. This greatly reduces the amount of acid in the stomach.

SE: Abdominal Pain, Headache, Diarrhea, Nausea/Vomiting, Clostridium difficile Diarrhea, Bone Fractures

DI: The most well-known drug interaction involving PPIs is probably the one between omeprazole/esomeprazole and clopidogrel. Clopidogrel must be activated by the enzyme CYP2C19 in order to be effective. Omeprazole and Esomeprazole (an isomer of omeprazole) inhibit CYP2C19. As a result, the effect (i.e. activity in preventing blood clots) of clopidogrel is reduced when used in conjunction with omeprazole or esomeprazole. Also, some drugs (e.g. levothyroxine) rely on stomach acid for optimal absorption. Since PPIs reduce stomach acid, absorption of other drugs can be impaired.

Notes: In patients with Clostridium difficile diarrhea (pseudomembranous colitis) use of proton pump inhibitors increases the chances that the Clostridium difficile infection will recur.

HISTAMINE-2 RECEPTOR ANTAGONISTS (H₂-BLOCKER)

Examples: Zantac® (ranitidine), Pepcid® (famotidine), Tagamet® (cimetidine), Axid® (nizatidine)

Indications: Gastroesophageal Reflux Disease (GERD), Peptic Ulcer Disease (PUD)

MoA: Histamine binds to receptors in the stomach that cause acid to be released from parietal cells. Histamine-2 (H2) blockers prevent histamine from binding to these receptors, thus preventing acid from being secreted into the stomach by parietal cells.

SE: Constipation, headache, seizures (rare), gynecomastia (with cimetidine only).

DI: Some drugs (e.g. levothyroxine) rely on stomach acid for optimal absorption. Since H2 blockers reduce stomach acid, absorption of other drugs can be impaired.

Examples: Tegretol® (carbamazepine), Trileptal® (oxcarbazepine), Topamax® (topiramate), Dilantin® (phenytoin), Neurontin® (gabapentin), Keppra® (levetiracetam), Lyrica® (pregabalin), Vimpat® (lincosamide), Depakote® (divalproex), Lamictal® (lamotrigine), Zonegran® (zonisamide)

Indications: Epilepsy/Seizures, Nerve Pain, Psychiatric Disorders

MoA: Anti-epileptic drugs work by essentially suppressing nerve activity. There are several specific mechanisms by which this effect is accomplished (e.g. sodium ion channel modulation, GABA* receptor stimulation, glutamate** receptor antagonism, benzodiazepine receptor stimulation).

SE: Drowsiness, mental slowing, skin rash, weight gain, liver toxicity, Stevens-Johnson Syndrome (rare), increased risk of suicidal thoughts and behavior.

DI: Nervous system suppression is greater when combined with other drugs that suppress the nervous system (e.g. benzodiazepines, opioids, alcohol).

Notes: *GABA (gamma-aminobutyric acid) is the primary inhibitory neurotransmitter of the central nervous system. ** Glutamate is the primary excitatory neurotransmitter of the central nervous system. Anti-epileptic drugs are also referred to as anticonvulsants.

Examples: Penicillin, Amoxicillin, Augmentin® (amoxicillin/clavulanate), Keflex® (cephalexin), Cipro® (ciprofloxacin), Avelox® (moxifloxacin), Levaquin® (levofloxacin), Flagyl® (metronidazole), Zithromax®/Z-pak® (azithromycin), Biaxin® (clarithromycin), Vancocin® (vancomycin), Zosyn® (piperacillin/tazobactam)

Indications: Bacterial Infections

MoA: There are several different antibiotics with several different mechanisms of action. On a basic level, they all work by exploiting differences between bacterial cells and human cells. For instance, clarithromycin (a macrolide antibiotic) works by binding to the 50S ribosomal subunit of bacterial ribosomes., resulting in inhibition of protein synthesis. Ultimately this protein synthesis inhibition kills the cell. Human cells remain unharmed because they do not have 50S ribosomal subunits in their ribosomes.

SE: Diarrhea

DI: Antibiotics increase the effect of warfarin, leading to an increased risk of bleeding in patients taking warfarin. Antibiotics also decrease the effect of oral contraceptives. Oral administration of certain antibiotics should be separated from antacids or multivitamins containing divalent or trivalent cations (e.g. Calcium (Ca^{2+}), Magnesium (Mg^{2+}), Iron (Fe^{2+}/Fe^{3+}), Aluminum (Al^{3+})) by at least 2 – 4 hours.

Examples: Ecotrin® (aspirin), Motrin® (ibuprofen), Aleve® (naproxen), Mobic® (meloxicam), Indocin® (indomethacin), Voltaren® (diclofenac), Celebrex® (celecoxib)

Indications: Pain, Fever, Rheumatoid Arthritis, Osteoarthritis

MoA: Cyclooxygenase (COX) is an enzyme that is involved in the creation of prostaglandins and thromboxane. Prostaglandins are chemical mediators of inflammation (i.e. they promote inflammation). Prostaglandins also play a role in protecting the gastric mucosa (the lining of the stomach). NSAIDs work by inhibiting COX. There are two subtypes of the cyclooxygenase enzyme (COX-1 and COX-2). Cyclooxygenase-1 is associated with normal physiologic functions (e.g. gastric mucosal protection and blood clotting) and COX-2 is associated with inflammation. Most NSAIDs are nonselective inhibitors of COX (i.e. they inhibit both subtypes, COX-1 and COX-2). Celecoxib is unique because it selectively inhibits COX-2. This is important since inhibition of COX-1 is associated with a higher incidence of gastric mucosal damage. As a result, celecoxib is less irritating to the stomach and less likely to cause or aggravate ulcers of the gastric mucosa compared to the other NSAIDs. Another drug that stands out from the crowd is aspirin. Aspirin is an *irreversible* inhibitor of COX, whereas the other NSAIDs are reversible inhibitors. This irreversible inhibition leads to a more profound antiplatelet effect (i.e. prevents blood from clotting more than any other NSAID), thus it is used in preventing heart attacks and strokes.

SE: Nausea, vomiting, renal impairment, GI ulceration, hypernatremia and heart failure (increased sodium retention causes increased water retention).

DI: Increased risk of bleeding (especially gastrointestinal bleeding) when used with other drugs that reduce blood clot formation (i.e. anticoagulants and antiplatelets such as warfarin, clopidogrel, dabigatran, and heparin). Increased risk of renal failure when used with other drugs that can impair renal function (e.g. ACE inhibitors, ARBs, diuretics).

Examples: Oxycontin® (oxycodone), MS Contin® (morphine) Dilaudid® (hydromorphone), codeine, hydrocodone

Indications: Pain

MoA: Agonist at opioid receptors, particularly mu (µ) opioid receptors. Mu (µ) opioid receptors are involved in pain and wakefulness – thus pain relief and sedation are associated with opioid drugs.

SE: Sedation, respiratory depression, constipation

DI: Increased incidence of sedation and respiratory depression when taken with other drugs that suppress the nervous system (e.g. benzodiazepines).

Notes: In patients using opioids on a long-term basis, the drugs must be discontinued gradually over time to avoid opioid withdrawal. In general, it is recommended that you decrease the dose by 25-50% per day. The patient should be monitored closely during discontinuation. If withdrawal symptoms appear, return to the previous dose and decrease more slowly or more gradually. Take note that constipation is the only side effect that patients do not gain a tolerance for.

****

Opioid Conversion

When converting from one opioid to another, it is safer (helps avoid dangerous side effects, like respiratory depression) to underestimate the equivalent dose, as opposed to overestimating. As a rule of thumb, begin with one-half of the estimated equivalent dose and provide the patient with a rescue supply for uncontrolled pain.

****

Examples: Ativan® (lorazepam), Klonopin® (clonazepam), Halcion® (triazolam), Versed® (midazolam), Onfi® (clobazam), Restoril® (temazepam), Prosom® (estazolam), Xanax® (alprazolam), Valium®/Diastat® (diazepam), Librium® (chlordiazepoxide), Tranxene® (clorazepate)

Indications: Insomnia, Anxiety, Agitation, Seizures, Muscle Spasms, Alcohol Withdrawal

MoA: Benzodiazepines bind to benzodiazepine receptors (BNZ_1 and BNZ_2), which enhances the effect of GABA (gamma-aminobutyric acid; the primary inhibitory (opposite of excitatory) neurotransmitter of the central nervous system). Specifically, BNZ_1 receptors stimulation promotes sleep and BNZ_2 receptor stimulation promotes muscle relaxation and inhibits memory function.

SE: Drowsiness/somnolence, headache, dizziness, confusion, fatigue

DI: Increased central nervous system depression when taken with other drugs that suppress the nervous system (e.g. non-benzodiazepine sedative-hypnotics, opioids, anticonvulsants, alcohol).

Notes: All drugs in this class are Schedule IV controlled substances.

NON-BENZODIAZEPINE SEDATIVE-HYPNOTICS

Examples: Ambien® (zolpidem), Lunesta® (eszopiclone), Sonata® (zaleplon)

Indications: Insomnia

MoA: Similar to benzodiazepines, but generally these drugs bind to BNZ_1 receptors (promote sleep) more than BNZ_2 receptors.

SE: Drowsiness/somnolence, headache, dizziness.

DI: Increased central nervous system depression when taken with other drugs that suppress the nervous system (e.g. benzodiazepines, opioids, anticonvulsants, alcohol).

Notes: All drugs in this class are Schedule IV controlled substances.

Combination drug are formulations containing two or more active ingredients. These are 20 commonly prescribed combination drugs that did not make the Top 210 Prescription Drugs list. I added them because they can be a real killer on the exam. After all, you either know them or you don't.

Aggrenox® (aspirin/dipyridamole) *Blood clot prevention*
Benicar® HCT (olmesartan/hydrochlorothiazide) *High blood pressure*
Benzaclin® (benzoyl peroxide/clindamycin) *Acne (topical)*
Fioricet® (acetaminophen/caffeine/butalbital) *Migraines and headaches*
Glucovance® (glyburide/metformin) *Diabetes*
Hyzaar® (losartan/hydrochlorothiazide) *High blood pressure*
Jalyn® (dutasteride/tamsulosin) *Enlarged prostate (BPH)*
Janumet® (sitagliptin/metformin) *Diabetes
Kaletra® (lopinavir/ritonavir) *HIV/AIDS*
Lotrel® (amlodipine/benazepril) *High blood pressure*
Metaglip® (glipizide/metformin) *Diabetes*
Sinemet® (carbidopa/levodopa) *Parkinson's disease*
Stalevo® (carbidopa/levodopa/entacapone) *Parkinson's disease*
Symbyax® (olanzapine/fluoxetine) *Depression in bipolar disorder*
Tenoretic® (atenolol/chlorthalidone) *High blood pressure*
Tobradex® (tobramycin/dexamethasone) *Bacterial infections of the eye*
Tribenzor® (olmesartan/amlodipine/hydrochlorothiazide) *High blood pressure*
Vicoprofen® (ibuprofen/hydrocodone) *Pain and inflammation*
Vimovo® (naproxen/esomeprazole) *Arthritis pain and stomach acid*
Zegerid® (omeprazole/sodium bicarbonate) *GERD*

Note: blood pressure medications are commonly formulated as combination drugs. This is because most patients with hypertension need more than one medication to achieve adequate blood pressure control.

What is the benefit of having two or more active ingredients in one capsule or tablet?

One of the biggest challenges prescribers and pharmacists face is getting patients to consistently take their medications exactly as prescribed. When a patient consistently remembers to take their medication as prescribed, the patient is considered to be *compliant* (or *"adherent"*). When the patient frequently misses doses of medication, the patient is considered to be *non-compliant* (or *"non-adherent"*). Patients may lack consistency due to forgetfulness, lack of education regarding the benefits of therapy, and/or an inability to afford the medication. By supplying two or more active ingredients in one capsule or tablet, the patient now only has to remember to take one tablet or capsule instead of two. This has a positive impact on patient compliance.

When trying to determine the drug class of a drug, sometimes you will find a clue in the drug name itself, particularly in the suffix. Below are some examples:

-olol = bet-blocker (e.g. metoprolol, atenolol, propranolol, bisoprolol) to lower blood pressure or treat other cardiac diseases such as arrhythmias.

-statin = HMG-CoA Reductase Inhibitor (e.g. atorvastatin, simvastatin, lovastatin, pravastatin) to lower cholesterol.

-sartan = angiotensin receptor blocker (ARB) (e.g. valsartan, losartan, olmesartan) to reduce blood pressure.

-isone = corticosteroid (e.g. prednisone, methylprednisone, hydrocortisone) to suppress the immune system.

-afil = phosphodiesterase 5 (PDE 5) inhibitor (e.g. tadalafil, sildenafil, vardenafil) to treat erectile dysfunction and pulmonary arterial hypertension.

-pril = angiotensin converting enzyme inhibitor (ACEI) (e.g. lisinopril, benazepril) to lower blood pressure.

-osin = alpha adrenergic receptor blocker (α-blocker) (e.g. doxazosin, terazosin, prazosin) to treat high blood pressure and benign prostatic hyperplasia (BPH).

-floxacin = fluoroquinolone antibiotic (e.g. ciprofloxacin, moxifloxacin, levofloxacin) to treat bacterial infections.

-icillin = penicillin antibiotic (e.g. penicillin, amoxicillin, ampicillin, methicillin) to treat bacterial infections.

Ceph- or **Cef-** = cephalosporin antibiotic (e.g. cephalexin, cefazolin, ceftriaxone, ceftazidime, cefdinir) to treat bacterial infections.

-azole = antifungal (e.g. clotrimazole, ketoconazole) to treat fungal infections.

-vir = antiviral (e.g. ritonavir, lopinavir, acyclovir, valacyclovir) to treat viral infections like shingles, genital herpes, and HIV/AIDS.

-prazole = proton pump inhibitor (PPI) (e.g. omeprazole, lansoprazole, pantoprazole, rabeprazole) to suppress stomach acid production.

-gliptin = dipeptidyl peptidase 4 (DPP-4) inhibitor (e.g. saxagliptin, sitagliptin, linagliptin) to lower blood sugar in type II diabetes mellitus.

-triptan = serotonin agonist (5-HT agonist) (e.g. sumatriptan, zolmitriptan, naratriptan, eletriptan) to treat migraine headaches.

-setron = 5-HT$_3$ (serotonin) antagonist (e.g. ondansetron, palonosetron, granisetron) to treat or prevent nausea and vomiting (especially nausea and vomiting associated with cancer chemotherapy).

-dronate = bisphosphonate (e.g. ibandronate, alendronate, risedronate) to treat or prevent osteoporosis.

-pam or **–lam** = benzodiazepine (e.g. alprazolam, clonazepam, oxazepam, diazepam) to treat anxiety and insomnia.

There are four major types of drug interactions: drug-drug, drug-supplement, drug-food, and drug-disease. Below you will find a list of the most common drug interactions.

Common Drug-Drug Interactions

Warfarin and NSAIDs*

Warfarin is an anticoagulant used to prevent or treat blood clots. A major side effect of warfarin is bleeding. NSAIDs are notorious for damaging the lining of the stomach, which has the potential to lead to a GI bleed. When warfarin and NSAIDs are used together, the risk of a life-threatening GI bleed increases significantly. NSAIDs also have some "anti-platelet" (blood-thinning) effect, which further increases bleed risk. *Some examples of generic NSAIDs include: Ibuprofen, Naproxen, Aspirin, Meloxicam, Indomethacin, and Diclofenac.

Warfarin and Antibiotics

Antibiotics increase the bleeding risk associated with warfarin. The reason for this is explained below.

How Warfarin Works
Vitamin K is used by the body to activate the "vitamin K-dependent clotting factors" (factors 2, 7, 9, and 10). Once vitamin K is used to activate a clotting factor, it is deactivated (incapable of activating more clotting factors) unless it is reactivated by the enzyme "Vitamin K Epoxide Reductase Complex 1" (VKORC1). Warfarin works by inhibiting VKORC1, thus preventing activation of vitamin K-dependent clotting factors. In simpler terms, warfarin reduces blood clotting by keeping vitamin K in its deactivated form. Since vitamin K is deactivated, it cannot activate certain clotting factors.

Why Antibiotics Interact with Warfarin
Vitamin K enters the body from *two sources*: the diet (e.g. green leafy vegetables, mayonnaise) **and** intestinal flora (normal bacteria that reside in the intestine). Intestinal flora produces vitamin K, which gets absorbed into the bloodstream. When antibiotics are introduced into the body, the intestinal flora gets killed off (to some degree). Since there are fewer bacteria producing vitamin K in the intestine, less vitamin K enters the bloodstream from that source. This results in an exaggerated effect of warfarin, potentially leading to over-anticoagulation and bleeding.

Oral Contraceptives [and] Antibiotics

Antibiotics (especially Rifampin) can decrease the effect of oral contraceptives, which increases the likelihood of contraceptive failure (increased risk of pregnancy). The prevailing theory behind this interaction is reduced enterohepatic circulation of estrogen caused by antibiotic-induced reduction of intestinal flora.

Enterohepatic Circulation of Estrogen

Typically some of the estrogen is eliminated by excretion into the bile (from ingestion the estrogen goes to the intestine, then the bloodstream, then the liver where some of it goes into the bile, which is dumped into the intestine to be eliminated during defecation. Some of the estrogen that goes into the bile gets hydrolyzed by intestinal flora and subsequently reabsorbed into the blood where it is given another opportunity to exert its pharmacologic effect. Since antibiotics kill of intestinal flora (to some degree), less estrogen gets hydrolyzed and reabsorbed (i.e. less estrogen gets recycled).

Nitrates [and] PDE-5 Inhibitors*

Both of these drugs dilate blood vessels. When taken together, blood pressure can drop to a dangerously low level. PDE-5 inhibitors include: Sildenafil, Vardenafil, and Tadalafil.

Common Drug-Supplement Interactions

St. John's Wort [and] CYP3A4 Substrates

St. John's Wort induces (increases) the enzyme CYP3A4, which is debatably the most important enzyme involved in drug metabolism involved in the metabolism of approximately 50% of all drugs. Induction of CYP3A4 leads to the deactivation of drugs that are substrates of CYP3A4 (i.e. rely on CYP3A4 for metabolism/elimination). Examples include oral contraceptives, HIV protease inhibitors, carbamazepine, colchicine, cyclosporine, corticosteroids (e.g. dexamethasone, methylprednisolone), and many others.

Garlic [and] CYP3A4 Substrates

Garlic has an effect similar to St. John's Wort - it induces CYP3A4.

Cations* [and] Levothyroxine, Quinolones, Tetracyclines, and Bisphosphonates

These drugs can chelate (i.e. bind to) <u>divalent cations</u> (e.g. magnesium (Mg^{2+}), calcium (Ca^{2+})) and <u>trivalent cations</u> (e.g. iron (Fe^{3+}), aluminum (Al^{3+})) in the gut, leading to precipitation (solidification) of the drug-ion complex. The precipitated drug never gets absorbed and passes through the GI tract, never getting the opportunity to exert its pharmacologic effect. *Only polyvalent cations (e.g. not Na^+, K^+). Remember a *cation* is a positively charged ion, and an *anion* is a negatively charged ion.

Ginkgo and NSAIDs, Anticoagulants, or Anti-platelets

Ginkgo has anti-platelet effects. When combined with other drugs that have an inhibitory effect on blood clotting, the risk of bleeding is increased. *Anti-platelets include drugs like clopidogrel and prasugrel.

Dong Quai and NSAIDs, Anticoagulants, or Anti-platelets

Dong Quai is primarily used to treat PMS, menstrual cramps, and symptoms of menopause. It contains chemicals known as "coumarin derivatives" (notice how the name "coumarin" is similar to Coumadin® (warfarin)). Coumarin derivatives, like warfarin, are vitamin K antagonists, so it is not surprising that dong quai increases the risk of bleeding when taken with other drugs that inhibit blood clotting.

Fish Oil and NSAIDs, Anticoagulants, or Anti-platelets

At doses greater than 3 grams/day, fish oil can increase the risk of bleeding. Not surprisingly, the risk of bleeding is significantly higher when fish oil is taken with other drugs that increase the risk of bleeding.

Common Drug-Food Interactions

HMG-CoA Reductase Inhibitors (Statins) and Grapefruit Juice

Grapefruit juice inhibits the enzyme CYP3A4, which is a major enzyme involved in the metabolism of certain statins (….). This causes the statin levels to be higher than normal, leading to increased risk of rhabdomyolysis.

Levodopa and Protein

Lovedopa is used for treating symptoms of Parkinson's Disease. Dietary protein (e.g. from meat, nuts, and dairy products) interferes with the intestinal absorption of levodopa. Proteins also interfere with levodopa crossing the blood-brain barrier (levodopa must cross this barrier to reach its site of action). As a result, when levodopa is taken with a high protein meal, less levodopa reaches the site of action (the brain).

Warfarin and Foods High in Vitamin K*

Since warfarin exerts its pharmacologic effect by interfering with the activity of vitamin K, the effect of warfarin can be decreased if there is an increase in dietary vitamin K. As a general rule, patients on warfarin should not avoid vitamin K, but they should make an effort to be consistent in how much vitamin K they consume each day. *Foods high in vitamin K include: Spinach, Kale, Collard Greens, Turnip Greens, Broccoli, Brussels Sprouts, Mayonnaise, Green Tea, and Canola Oil, and Others.
Note: Be aware that *some* vitamin supplements contain vitamin K.

Monoamine Oxidase Inhibitors (MAOIs)* and Foods/Beverages Rich in Tyramine*
Tyramine is a monoamine that stimulates catecholamine release in the body. Catecholamines (e.g. epinephrine, norepinephrine) are vasopressors (increase blood pressure). When the enzyme monoamine oxidase is inhibited (e.g. by MAOIs), tyramine does not get eliminated. As a result, tyramine builds up as it is consumed, leading to massive release of catecholamines and hypertensive crisis (potentially fatal). *Foods/beverages rich in tyramine include the following examples: most things that are smoked, aged, pickled, or fermented (e.g. aged cheeses, aged meats, wines), chocolate, licorice, tofu, soy sauce, avocados, and bananas. *Monoamine Oxidase Inhibitors (MAOIs) include the following examples: Tranylcypromine, Phenelzine, and Selegiline.

Common Drug-Disease Interactions

Aspirin and Peptic Ulcer Disease
Aspirin has an anti-platelet effect (predisposes patients to bleeding) and damages the lining of the stomach. Peptic ulcers are lesions in the lining of the stomach. Connect the dots.

NSAIDs and Chronic Renal Failure
NSAIDs decrease prostaglandin production. Prostaglandins promote renal blood flow. Less prostaglandin leads to less renal blood flow. Less blood flow leads to additional renal impairment.

TCAs* and Dementia
Tricyclic antidepressants (TCAs) have anti-cholinergic effects. Dementia is theorized to result from an imbalance (relatively low acetylcholine) between two neurotransmitters (acetylcholine and dopamine). When a patient with dementia takes a drug with anti-cholinergic properties, the dementia can get worse.

Solution – made up of a solute and a solvent; the solute molecules dissolve into a homogenous, single-phase mixture with the solvent.

Syrup – Highly concentrated water-based sugar solutions.
Example: Simple Syrup (85%(w/v) solution of sucrose in water).

Elixir – Solutions containing water, alcohol, and sweetener.
Example: Lortab® Elixir.

Tincture – Usually alcoholic extracts of crude materials.
Example: Tincture of opium is derived from the poppy plant (*Papaver somniferum*) – a crude (i.e. raw) material.

Suspension – a mixture of particles (could be solid or fluid) dispersed in a fluid; the particles do not dissolve, the mixture is two-phase.*

Emulsion – a suspension of two immiscible *liquids* (two liquids that will not dissolve in one another as they would in a solution).
Example: Oil in water.

*Two-phase mixtures (e.g. suspensions/emulsions) must be shaken (you should put a label on the prescription bottle that says "shake well") to ensure that the patient is receiving the correct amount of medication in each dose. For instance, look at the image below. Imagine that the drug is represented by the gray phase. If the mixture is not shaken, the patient will receive too little of the gray phase (the drug) in the first few doses and too much of the gray phase (the drug) in the last few doses.

Illustration: *Why Suspensions Must Be Shaken*

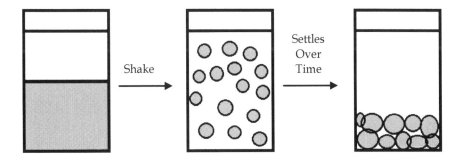

Tablets
A powdery mixture of an active pharmaceutical ingredient and excipients (inert/inactive ingredients, sometimes referred to as "fillers") pressed into a disc or other small shape. Many, if not most, drugs are available in tablet form.

Capsules
Capsules are basically made up of two parts: the shell (usually made of gelatin or cellulose) and the contents (may be drug powder, pellets, small tablets, or liquid). Many drugs are available in capsule form

Caplets
Caplets are basically capsule-shaped tablets.

Enteric Coated (EC) Tablets
These are tablets coated with a special material (enteric coating) that will not dissolve at a low pH (i.e. in the acidic environment of the stomach), but will dissolve at a higher pH (i.e. in the small intestine). As a result, when enteric coated tablets are ingested, they do not dissolve until they reach the intestine. This type of coating is typically used for medications that can irritate the lining of the stomach. A great example is enteric coated aspirin.

Sublingual (SL) Tablets
These tablets dissolve under the tongue and deliver the drug across the tissue beneath the tongue and directly into the bloodstream. By entering the bloodstream directly, the drug can exert is pharmacologic effect much more quickly. This method of administration also avoids first-pass metabolism (see section on routes of administration for further detail on first-pass metabolism). A great example is the nitroglycerin sublingual tablet.

Orally Disintegrating Tablets (ODT)
These are tablets that dissolve in the saliva. No water is required when taking an ODT. They are especially useful in patients that experience difficulty or pain when swallowing. For example, let's say a patient has experienced severe nausea and vomiting. The stomach acid from the vomit has damaged the lining of the patient's esophagus making it extremely painful to swallow. To avoid swallowing, the patient can use an ondansetron ODT (used to treat nausea) instead of the regular ondansetron tablets.

How do you determine that a generic drug is equivalent to a brand drug?
It is listed as an A-rated drug in the Federal Orange Book.

What is the official title for the Orange Book?
"Approved Drug Products with Therapeutic Equivalence Evaluations."

True or false. A drug with a narrow therapeutic index is never considered to be generically equivalent to the brand name product.
True.

A prescription For Lipitor® is given to you verbally over the telephone. Should you dispense brand Lipitor or the generic equivalent atorvastatin?
Atorvastatin. You would only dispense the brand name if the prescriber (or his/her agent) expressly said that the brand name is necessary and substitution is not allowed.

What is the definition of a narrow therapeutic index drug?
A drug that requires careful titration and patient monitoring in order to achieve safe and effective use, and one of the two following criteria must apply:
- There is less than a 2-fold difference between the median lethal dose (LD50) and the median effective dose (ED50).
- There is less than a 2-fold difference between the minimum toxic concentration and the minimum effective concentration.

Note: ED50 is the dose that produces the desired effect in 50% of the population using the drug, and LD 50 is the dose that is lethal in 50% of the population using the drug.

Does the FDA publish a current list of NTI drugs?
No.

NDC stands for "National Drug Code." An NDC number is an 11-digit numbers divided into 3 parts. They identify <u>who</u> manufactured the product, <u>what</u> the product is, and usually the <u>size</u> of the package the product comes in. The format of an NDC number is as follows:
NDC Number structure
12345–1234–12

First Segment (5 digits)
The first 5 number segment of the NDC number identifies the manufacturer of a product (e.g. 00093 is the 5-digit code for TEVA, 52544 represents Watson).

Second Segment (4 digits)
The middle 4 number segment of the NDC number identifies the product made by the manufacturer (e.g. 0913 is Watson's 4-digit code for Norco® 3/325 mg).

Third Segment (2 digits)
The final 2 number segment of the NDC number usually identifies the package size of the product (e.g. The NDC number for a 100 tablet bottle of Watson's Norco® 5/325 mg is 52544-0913-01 and the NDC number for a 500 tablet bottle is 52544-0913-05).

> <u>Note</u>: frequently, one of the trailing zeroes is omitted from the NDC number displayed on the label of the manufacturer's stock bottle. For instance, the 11-digit NDC 00093-0287-01 would typically be displayed on the stock bottle in one of the following three forms:
>
> 0093-0287-01
> 00093-287-01
> 00093-0287-1

Which drugs get assigned a lot number?
All drug products are assigned a lot number by the manufacturer. A different lot number is assigned to each batch of drug. So, all drugs within the same batch share the same lot number.

What is the purpose of the lot number?
Lot numbers play an indispensible role in drug manufacturing. If there is an abnormality with a drug product, such as discoloration or contamination, only the affected batch has to be recalled.

What would happen if there were no lot numbers (or nothing conceptually similar)?
During a recall, drug products lacking a lot number must be treated like they were in the affected batch. So, without lot numbers to identify which batch a drug belongs to, just one problem with one bottle of a drug could necessitate the recall of all batches of the drug.

Do all prescription drugs have an expiration date?
Yes, the FDA requires manufacturers to assign expiration dates for all prescription drugs.

Do expiration dates mean anything? Are they truly important?
Yes, the expiration date is the final date through which the manufacturer can guarantee the potency and safety of the drug.

If the label on a drug indicates the expiration date is 08/2018, is the drug considered expired in 08/02/2018?
No, the drug would be considered expired on the first day after 08/2018, which would be 09/01/2013.

The day is July 19, 2015. The expiration date on a vial of insulin is 09/31/2016. The stopper of the insulin vial was first punctured for use on June 18, 2015. The insulin will be expired after which day?
A. 06/18/2015
B. 07/16/2013
C. 07/18/2013
D. 09/31/2016

> **Answer:**
> B. 07/16/2015
> Since the expiration date printed on the vial is 09/31/2016, the rubber stopper of the vial may be first punctured for use up to 09/31/2016; however, once punctured the contents of the vial only remain sterile for 28 days.

Class I Recalls
A recall is categorized as class I if there is a reasonable probability that use of (or exposure to) the recalled product will cause <u>serious adverse health consequences up to and including death</u>.

Class II Recalls
A recall is categorized as class II if there is a possibility that use of (or exposure to) the recalled product could cause <u>temporary or medically reversible adverse health consequences</u>.

Class III Recalls
A recall is categorized as class III if use of the recalled product is <u>unlikely to cause adverse health consequences</u>.

Review Question:
What is the most serious class of FDA recall?
Class I recall.

What temperature range must be maintained in a <u>freezer</u> where drugs are stored?
-25°C to -10°C (or -13F to 14°F)

What temperature range must be maintained for drugs stored in a <u>cold</u> environment?
2°C to 8°C (or 36°F to 46°F)

What temperature range must be maintained for drugs stored in a <u>cool</u> environment?
8°C to 15°C (or 46°F to 59°F)

What temperature range must be maintained for drugs stored at <u>room temperature</u>?
20°C to 25°C (or 68°F to 77°F)

What temperature range must be maintained for drugs stored in a <u>warm</u> environment?
30°C to 40°C (or 86°F to 104°F)

How do you define <u>excessive heat</u>?
Temperatures > 40°C (or > 104°F)

How do you define <u>dry place</u>?
Average relative humidity = or < 40%

State Board of Pharmacy
Each state has its own board of pharmacy which is responsible for protecting the health, safety, and welfare of its citizens in pharmacy-related matters. This is accomplished through the enforcement of state pharmacy laws and regulations.

Food and Drug Administration (FDA)
The FDA enforces drug manufacturing laws and regulates prescription drug advertising, which is known as "direct to consumer" (DTC) advertising.

Drug Enforcement Agency (DEA)
The DEA enforces of the Federal Controlled Substance Act, and determines which drugs are placed on the federal controlled substance schedule.

Occupational Safety and Health Administration (OSHA)
OSHA enforces health and safety laws. The most important topic OSHA deals with in pharmacy is minimizing the risk of employee exposure to bloodborne pathogens. This is particularly relevant to pharmacies that compound infusions and pharmacies that provide vaccinations.

Federal Trade Commission (FTC)
The FTC is in charge of regulating advertisement of OTC drugs, medical devices, cosmetics, and foods.
> Note: Vitamins and herbal supplements are considered "foods" in the eyes of the law.

What is a "misbranded" drug?

Many things can be construed as misbranding. Below is a list of some examples of misbranding:

- False or misleading labeling.
- Not compliant with packaging/labeling requirements.
- Unclear wording is present on the label.
- Inadequate directions for use.
- Drug use poses a danger if used as prescribed.
- Generic name is not displayed in font at least half as large as the brand name font.

What is an "adulterated" drug?

A drug that has a quality, strength, or purity that is different from what is stated on the label.

What characteristics define each schedule of controlled substances?

Schedule I Controlled Substance (e.g. GHB, Heroin)
- High abuse potential.
- No accepted medical use.
- Lacks safety.

Schedule II Controlled Substance (e.g. Morphine, Codeine)
- High potential for abuse.
- Accepted medical use.
- Severe potential for physical/psychological dependence.

Schedule III Controlled Substance (e.g. Testosterone, Dronabinol)
- Moderate abuse potential.
- Accepted medical use.
- Moderate-low potential for dependence.

Schedule IV Controlled Substance (e.g. Diazepam, Modafinil)
- Mild abuse potential.
- Accepted medical use.
- Mild potential for physical/psychological dependence.

Schedule V Controlled Substance
- Low abuse potential.
- Accepted medical use.
- Low potential for physical/psychological dependence.

It is important to be able to recognize which schedule a controlled substance belongs to. Below, I have listed the names of some common controlled substances according to the schedule in which they belong.

Schedule I Controlled Substances

- GHB (gamma hydroxybutyric acid)
- Heroin
- LSD (lysergic acid diethylamide)
- Marijuana
- MDMA (3, 4-methylenedioxymethamphetamine)
- Psilocybin (hallucinogenic found in certain mushrooms)

Schedule II Controlled Substances

C-II Opioids:
- codeine
- Duragesic® (fentanyl)
- Dilaudid®, Exalgo® (hydromorphone)
- Dolophine®, Methadose® (methadone)
- MS Contin®, Kadian® (morphine)
- Roxicodone®, Oxycontin® (oxycodone)
- Opana® (oxymorphone)
- Sufenta® (sufentanil)

C-II Stimulants:
- Adderall® (amphetamine/dextroamphetamine)
- cocaine
- Desoxyn® (methamphetamine)
- Concerta®, Metadate®, Methylin®, Ritalin® (methylphenidate)

C-II Depressants:
- Amytal® (amobarbital)
- Nembutal® (pentobarbital)
- phencyclidine (PCP)
- Seconal® (secobarbital)

C-II Hallucinogens:
- Cesamet® (Nabilone)

Schedule III Controlled Substances

C-III Opioids:
- Buprenex®, Subutex® (buprenorphine)
- Suboxone® (buprenorphine/naloxone)
- Paregoric® (camphorated tincture of opium)
-

The following opioids are considered C-III when used in limited quantities *in combination with other medications*.
- codeine (e.g. Tylenol #3, which is mixed with acetaminophen)
- morphine
- opium

C-III Mixed Opioid Agonist/Antagonists:
- nalorphine

C-III Stimulants:
- Didrex®, Regimex (benzphetamine)
- Bontril® (phendimetrazine)

C-III Depressants:
- barbituric acid and its derivatives
- Ketalar® (ketamine)

These otherwise Schedule II depressants are considered Schedule III when they exist in a compound, mixture, or suppository
- amobarbital
- pentobarbital
- secobarbital

C-III Anabolic Steroids:
All anabolic steroids are C-III
- AndroGel®, Testim®, Axiron®, Depo-Testosterone® (testosterone)
- Pregnyl®, Novarel® (chorionic gonadotropin)
- Oxandrin® (oxandrolone)

C-III Hallucinogens:
- Marinol® (dronabinol)

Schedule IV Controlled Substances

C-IV Depressants (Benzodiazepines):
Note: All prescription benzodiazepines are classified as Schedule C-IV. The best way to recognize a benzodiazepine is by the last part of the generic name of the dug. The generic drug name almost always ends in "-pam" or "- lam." Below is a list of benzodiazepines. Exceptions to the naming rule are described.

- Xanax® (alprazolam)
- Librium® (chlordiazepoxide)
    o The first benzodiazepine formally discovered
    o The only benzodiazepine that ends in -epoxide.
    o The best way to tell by the name that this drug is a benzodiazepine is by the -diazep- in the name.
- Klonopin® (clonazepam)
- Tranxene® (clorazepate)
    o One of two benzodiazepines that end in -ate.
    o The -aze- is another way to tell by the name that this drug is a benzodiazepine.
- Valium®, Diastat® (diazepam)
- Prosom® (estazolam)
- Dalmane® (flurazepam)
- Ativan® (lorazepam)
- Versed® (midazolam)
- Restoril® (temazepam)

C-IV Depressants:
- Lunesta® (eszopiclone)
- Sonata® (zaleplon)
- Ambien® (zolpidem)
- phenobarbital

C-IV Mixed Opioid Agonist/Antagonists:
- Stadol® (butorphanol)
- Talwin® (pentazocine)

C-IV Stimulants:
- Provigil® (modafinil)
- Adipex-P®, Suprenza® (phentermine)
- Qsymia® (phentermine/topiramate)
- Meridia® (sibutramine)

Schedule V Controlled Substances

<u>C-V Opioids:</u>
*When the strength per unit dose is very small, these medications are classified as Schedule V.
- codeine
- Lomotil® (diphenoxylate/atropine)
- opium

True or false. Schedule I controlled substances can be dispensed pursuant to a valid, hand-signed prescription.
False, Schedule I controlled substances have no accepted medical use and cannot be prescribed.

In what setting might you find Schedule I controlled substances?
The only place Schedule I controlled substances can be legally utilized is in a legitimate research laboratory registered with the DEA to use Schedule I controlled substances.

True or false. Schedule II controlled substance prescription records can be stored in the same file as other prescription medications.
False, Schedule II prescription records must be stored separately from all other prescription records.

After an initial inventory of controlled substances has been taken (e.g. when the pharmacy first opens for business), how frequently must an inventory of controlled substances be taken?
At least every two years.

When taking an inventory of controlled substances, does the law require you to account for drug samples?
Yes, drug samples that contain controlled substances must be accounted for in the inventory record.

According to the federal controlled substance act (CSA), how should you store Schedule III – V prescription files?
Either separately from all other prescription records, or in such a way that they are readily retrievable from the non-controlled prescription records (e.g. Schedule III – V prescription records can be stored along with non-controlled substance prescription records if each controlled substance prescription is marked with the letter "C" in red ink).

When Schedule II controlled substances are sent to a reverse distributor because they are expired, damaged, or otherwise unusable, what form should be used?
DEA Form 222.

Who would be responsible for filling out the Form 222?
The reverse distributor – the entity receiving the substance is always the one that fills out the form.

When Schedule III – V controlled substances are returned, is a DEA Form 222 necessary?
No, Schedule III – V controlled substances may be transferred via invoice (DEA Form 222 is only used for Schedule I and II controlled substances).

How long must the pharmacy keep controlled substance return records, prescription records, and inventory records?
2 years.

Controlled Substance Prescription Requirements

What information must be included on a controlled substance prescription?
1. Patient's full name
2. Patient's address
3. Prescriber's full name
4. Prescribers work address
5. Prescriber's DEA number
6. Drug name
7. Drug strength
8. Dosage form
9. Quantity prescribed
10. Directions for use
11. Number of refills authorized (if any)

True or false. Federal law prohibits e-prescribing of C-II drugs.
False, federal law permits e-prescribing of C-II through C-V drugs; however, most state laws are currently stricter and place limitations on e-prescribing of controlled substances.

According to federal law, C-II prescriptions must be filled within how many days after being signed by the prescriber?
Federal law places no time limit within which a C-II prescription must be filled (i.e. the prescription is considered legally valid for an unlimited period of time after it is issued). Note, however, that certain states may have laws that do set time limits.

True or false. For controlled substance prescriptions, the maximum quantity that can be dispensed according to federal law is a 30-days' supply.
False, although some states and many insurance carriers limit controlled substance quantities to a 30-days' supply, there are no specific federal limits.
> Note: Remember that when federal and state laws differ, you must follow the stricter of the two laws.

Are verbal/oral orders (i.e. called in by the prescriber, no prescriber-signed prescription hard copy) for C-II prescriptions permitted?
Only in emergency situations (determined by the pharmacist).
Note: quantity prescribed must be limited to the amount adequate to treat the patient for the duration of the emergency period.

After calling in an emergency C-II prescription, what must the prescriber do next?
Provide the pharmacy with a written and signed hard copy, which the pharmacy files away with the verbal order.

When emergency C-II prescriptions are called in, a prescriber has how many days to furnish the pharmacy with a written and signed prescription?
7 days according to federal law (state laws may be stricter, depending on the state).

True or false. Refills for C-II prescriptions are legally permitted up to 5 refills in 6 months.
False, refills for C-II prescriptions are legally prohibited.

Are C-II prescriptions received by facsimile (fax machine) considered valid?
A pharmacy can use a faxed copy of a C-II prescription to fill a prescription, but *before* that prescription can be *dispensed* the original signed prescription must be presented to the pharmacist.

There are three exceptions which allow for C-II facsimile prescriptions to serve as the original prescription, what are they?
1. The prescription is being compounded for home infusion.
2. The prescription is for a patient in a long-term care facility.
3. The prescription is for a patient enrolled in a hospice care program.

A patient presents 6 prescriptions for Adderall 5 mg. Each prescription is written for 30 tablets with the instructions to take 1 tablet by mouth every morning and 1 tablet by mouth every afternoon at 3 PM. The situation appears suspicious since the patient has 6 prescriptions for Adderall. Is it even legal for the patient to have this many prescriptions for a C-II drug?
While it may be worth verifying the prescriptions with the prescriber before dispensing, a prescriber is legally entitled to issue a patient multiple C-II prescriptions as long as the total days' supply does not exceed 90 days, assuming the issuance of multiple prescriptions is permissible under applicable state laws.

> Note: these prescriptions would need to have the earliest fill date written on them (e.g. they would have to say "do not fill until 4/15," "do not fill until 4/30," etc.), they cannot all be filled at the same time.

Prescriptions for C-III, C-IV, and C-V controlled substances can be issued by what means?
- Orally.
- In writing.
- By facsimile.
- Electronically (e-prescribing) where state laws permit.

Are refills legally permissible for C-III, C-IV, and C-V prescriptions?
Yes, for C-III and C-IV drugs there can be up to 5 refills within 6 months of the date issued. Refill limitations do not apply for C-V prescriptions.

For non-controlled substance prescriptions, a prescriber's agent (e.g. nurse or secretary) may call in a verbal prescription. Is a prescriber's agent allowed to call in Schedule III – V prescriptions?
No, the individual prescriber must personally make the call to submit a C-III through V prescription verbally.

Is the individual prescriber required to personally send the fax when a C-III through V prescription is being submitted by facsimile?
No, faxes for C-III through V prescriptions may be sent by a prescriber's agent.

Can a prescriber post-date a prescription for a controlled substance (e.g. record the date of issuance as 8/14 when he/she actually wrote the prescription in 8/12)?
No. The prescriber might try to do this when he/she doesn't want the patient to have the prescription filled until 8/14, but the proper approach is to record the written date as 8/12 and write on the face of the prescription "do not fill until 8/14."

Can a controlled substance be delivered or shipped to an individual in another country if there is a valid prescription for the substance?
No, this type of exportation of a controlled substance is prohibited by the federal controlled substance act.

Prescribers that want to prescribe Schedule III – V controlled substances for treatment of narcotic addiction (i.e. buprenorphine drug products) must display what piece of additional information on the face of the prescription?
Their unique DEA registration identification number that begins with an "X" must be displayed, which is granted to prescribers that have obtained the necessary waiver* from the DEA (in addition to their standard DEA registration number).

> *Typically, controlled substances used to treat narcotic addiction can only be prescribed, administered, and/or dispensed within a Narcotic Treatment Facility (NTF), but the DEA can grant a waiver to a prescriber to allow him/her to prescribe, administer, and/or dispense C-III through V drugs for treatment of narcotic addiction outside of a NTF.

What should be done in the event that theft or loss of a controlled substance is discovered?
The DEA should be notified upon discovery and a DEA Form 106 should be filled out to document the theft or loss.

Summary of Federal Controlled Substance Act Requirements

	Schedule II	Schedule III & IV	Schedule V
DEA Registration	Required	Required	Required
Receiving Records	DEA Form-222	Invoices, Readily Retrievable	Invoices, Readily Retrievable
Prescriptions	Written Prescription*	Written, Oral, or Faxed Prescriptions	Written, Oral, Faxed, or Over The Counter**
Refills	No	No more than 5 within 6 months	As authorized when prescription is issued
Distribution Between Registrants	DEA Form-222	Invoices	Invoices
Theft or Significant Loss	Report and complete DEA Form 106	Report and complete DEA Form 106	Report and complete DEA Form 106

Note: All records must be maintained for 2 years, unless a state requires longer.
* Emergency prescriptions require a signed follow-up prescription. Exceptions: facsimile prescription serves as the original prescription when issued to residents of Long Term Care Facilities, Hospice patients, or compounded IV (i.e. Home Infusion) narcotic medications.
** Where authorized by state controlled substances authority.

What is the DEA Form 224 used for?
Applying for pharmacy DEA registration.

How frequently does a pharmacy's DEA registration need to be renewed?
Every 3 years.

What is the DEA Form 222 used for?
Ordering Schedule I and Schedule II controlled substances.

If you make a mistake when filling out a DEA Form 222 can you just cross out the error?
No, if an error is made then all copies of the 222 form must be voided and retained in your records.

How many carbon copies are attached to a DEA Form 222?
2 copies, so you have the original plus 2 copies.

What color is each copy of a DEA Form 222?
- The first page (original) is brown.
- The second page (first carbon copy) is green.
- The third page (second carbon copy) is blue.

When ordering Schedule II drugs for your pharmacy, what do you do with the first two pages (brown and green) of the DEA Form 222?
Give them to the supplier without separating them. For the form to be valid from the supplier's perspective, the brown and green copies must be intact with the carbon paper between them.

Which part of the DEA Form 222 is the supplier required to retain?
The first page (brown copy).

Which part of the DEA Form 222 does the supplier forward to the DEA?
The second page (green copy).

Which part of the DEA Form 222 is the pharmacy required to retain?
The third page (blue copy).

How long are you required to maintain records of your 222 forms?
2 years.

What is the DEA Form 222a used for?
Ordering more DEA 222 Forms.

What is the DEA Form 106 used for?
Reporting loss or theft of controlled substances.

What is the DEA Form 104 used for?
Closing a pharmacy/surrendering a pharmacy permit.

What is the DEA Form 41 used for?
Reporting the destruction of controlled substances.

Doctor of Medicine (MD)
Doctor of Osteopathic Medicine (DO)
Doctor of Dental Medicine (DMD)
Doctor of Dental Surgery (DDS)
Doctor of Optometry (OD)
Doctor of Podiatric Medicine (DPM)
Doctor of Veterinary Medicine (DVM)
Physician Assistant (PA)
Nurse Practitioner (NP)

Do pharmacists have prescribing authority?

In some states (e.g. New Mexico, North Carolina, Montana), pharmacists can obtain the authority to initiate medication therapy. Many other states allow pharmacists to have more limited prescriptive authority. Check with your state board of pharmacy to find out what the rules are in your state.

Can dentists prescribe medications to treat depression?

No, prescribers cannot prescribe medications to treat conditions outside of their scope of practice. For instance, a DVM cannot prescribe medications for a human, a DPM cannot prescribe medications to treat conditions of the eye, an OD cannot prescribe medications to treat conditions of the foot, etc.

> Note: In some states, other healthcare professionals may have prescriptive authority (e.g. certified nurse-midwives). Check with your state board of pharmacy.

How do I know if a prescriber's DEA number is valid?
There are two components of a DEA number, the letters and the numbers. First we will look at the letters.

The 1ST Letter
DEA numbers begin with 2 letters. The 1st letter of the DEA number provides information about the type of practitioner or registrant.
- A, B, or F for physicians, dentists, veterinarians, hospitals, and pharmacies.
- M for midlevel practitioners.
- P or R for drug distributors.

Note: The DEA number will start with an X for prescribers who have been granted a DEA waiver to write prescriptions for Subutex® or Suboxone® outside of a narcotic treatment program.

The 2ND Letter
The second letter of the DEA number will be the same as the first letter of the prescriber's last name or the first letter in the name of the business.

Now that you know what the letters in a DEA number represent, let's look at the equation to verify a DEA number using the numbers.

Part 1
Add the 2ND, 4TH, and 6TH digits of the DEA number and multiply the sum by 2 to get X.

Note: Remember to multiply the correct set of numbers by 2 (the 2ND, 4TH, and 6TH digits of the DEA number). If you add the 1ST, 3RD, and 5TH digits of the DEA number and multiply that sum by 2, you will get the wrong answer. This is probably the most common mistake people make.

Part 2
Add the 1ST, 3RD, and 5TH digits of the DEA number to get Y.

Part 3
Take your answer from Part 1 and add it to your answer from Part 2 to get Z. In other words, $X + Y = Z$.

Part 4
Your answer from part 3 (Z) will be a 2 digit number. If the DEA number is valid, then the second digit of your two digit answer from Part 3 (Z) will match the 7TH and final digit of the DEA number. For example, let's say your answer from Part 3 was Z = 4_8_. If the DEA number was valid, then the DEA number would end with an 8.

Practice Problem
Verify the example DEA number below.

John Smith, MD
DEA # FS8524616

Solution:
- The registrant is a physician (MD), so the first letter is A, B, or F.
- The prescriber's last name is Smith, so the second letter is S.
- 5 + 4 + 1 = 10 and 10 x 2 = 20... 8 + 2 + 6 = 16
- The sum of 20 and 16 is 36.
- The last number of the DEA number is 6, which is the same as the last number in the sum of 20 + 16.
- According to our analysis, this DEA number appears to be valid.

Note: The Drug Addiction Treatment Act of 2000 (DATA 2000) is the name of the law that requires prescribers to include their special DEA number (starting with "X") on prescriptions written for Subutex® or Suboxone®.

What is the purpose of the Health Insurance Portability and Accountability Act of 1996 (HIPAA)?
To protect the privacy of individual health information (referred to in the law as "protected health information" or "PHI").

If an individual's PHI has been breached, what must be done according to HIPAA?
The individual must be notified by the person or entity holding the information that their PHI was exposed. This is known as the "HIPAA Breach Notification Rule."

Does HIPAA set standards for protecting *electronic* PHI, such as electronic medical records (EMR)?
Yes.

When using or disclosing PHI, what principle should you keep in mind?
The principle of "minimum necessary use and disclosure."

"Minimum necessary use and disclosure" does not apply to certain situations, which include:
- Disclosures to a healthcare provider for treatment.
- Disclosures to the patient upon request.
- Disclosures authorized by the patient.
- Disclosures necessary to comply with other laws.
- Disclosures to the Dept. of Health and Human Services (HHS) for a compliance investigation, review, or enforcement.

How did the Omnibus Reconciliation Act of 1990 (OBRA '90) change pharmacy practice?
By requiring drug utilization reviews (DUR) and pharmaceutical care (i.e. pharmacist counseling) for Medicaid patients.

If OBRA '90 only requires an offer for pharmacist counseling to be made to Medicaid patients, why does *every* customer (including non-Medicaid customers) receive the same offer?
The "offer to counsel" became part of standard pharmacy business practices to ensure that all customers were receiving the same level of service.

How did the Poison Prevention Packaging Act of 1970 change the way we dispense drugs?
This act required drugs to be dispensed in child-resistant packaging (there are several exceptions; one exception is nitroglycerin sublingual tablets).

Why are nitroglycerin sublingual tablets exempt from the PPPA?
Nitroglycerin sublingual tablets are used to restore blood flow to the heart during an exacerbation of angina (characterized by acute chest pain), potentially preventing a myocardial infarction (heart attack). Child resistant packaging may cause an individual on the verge of a heart attack to struggle with opening the container of this potentially life-saving medication (nitroglycerin). As a result, this medication is exempt from the rules of the PPPA.

What is the intent of the PPPA?
The PPPA is intended to protect children from serious injury or illness caused by handling, using, or ingesting medications and certain household substances.

How is this accomplished?
The PPPA protects children by requiring manufacturers to use packaging that is *significantly difficult* for children under the age of 5 years old to open, yet not difficult for normal adults to open.

Pseudoephedrine can only be purchased from what location?
Behind the pharmacy counter or from a locked cabinet stored away from customers.

True or false. Pseudoephedrine can be purchased without a photo ID.
False.

What packaging requirement applies to solid oral dosage forms of pseudoephedrine?
They must be packaged and sold in blister packs, pseudoephedrine can never be sold as loose tablets/capsules.

Daily sales of pseudoephedrine are limited to what amount?
3.6 grams/day.

Monthly (30-day) sales of pseudoephedrine are limited to what amount?
9 grams/30 days.

Federal law limits the amount of pseudoephedrine purchased via mail order to what amount over a 30-day period?
7.5 grams.

What information must be logged during the sale of products containing pseudoephedrine?

- Product name.
- Quantity sold.
- Name and address of purchaser.
- Date and time of sale.
- Signature of purchaser.

Records from pseudoephedrine sales must be kept for what length of time?
2 years.

All medications have benefits (the intended therapeutic effect) and risks (side effects). Some drugs have higher risks than others. Those drugs with an unacceptably high level of risk typically do not reach the market or, if they have already reached the market, get withdrawn from the market (e.g. Vioxx®). What do you do when you have a medication with a very high level of risk that has a tremendous benefit for some patients? The answer is - restricted drug programs (also referred to as "REMS"). REMS is an acronym for Risk Evaluation and Mitigation Strategies. The FDA, pursuant to the FDA Amendments Act of 2007, can *require* manufacturers to comply with REMS to manage the risks associated with certain drugs. REMS are meant to ensure that the benefits of using a particular medication outweigh the associated risks.

What consequence can a manufacturer face for failing to comply with REMS?
A fine of at least $250,000 per incident.

Can manufacturers require its own REMS program without being required by the FDA to create such a program?
Yes.

Approximately how many drugs have a REMS program?
Over 100 drugs.

What are some of the most well-known and frequently used REMS programs?
iPLEDGE™, THALIDOMID REMS™., T.I.P.S., and Clozaril® National Registry.

What is iPLEDGE™?
iPLEDGE™ is a REMS program aimed at ensuring patients beginning isotretinoin therapy are not pregnant and preventing pregnancy in patients receiving isotretinoin therapy. Why? When used during pregnancy, isotretinoin has been clearly linked to severe birth defects.

> Note: several brand name formulations of isotretinoin are available: Absorbica®, Accutane®, Amnesteem®, Claravis®, Myorisan®, Sotret®, and Zenatane®.

THALIDOMID REMS™ (formerly known as S.T.E.P.S. ®)
THALIDOMID REMS™ was previously known as S.T.E.P.S.® (System for Thalidomide Education and Prescribing Safety). Thalomid® (thalidomide) can be used for the treatment of multiple myeloma and erythema nodosum leprosum, but the drug causes severe birth defects in unborn babies and venous thromboembolic events (deep vein thrombosis and pulmonary thromboembolism) in patients using the drug. Similar to isotretinoin, thalidomide can never be used in women who are pregnant or may become pregnant.

154

T.I.P.S.

Tikosyn In Pharmacy System (T.I.P.S.) is a REMS program aimed at communicating the risk of induced arrhythmia with the use of Tikosyn® (dofetilide). Tikosyn® (dofetilide) is used to induce and maintain normal cardiac sinus rhythm in highly symptomatic patients with atrial fibrillation or atrial flutter of more than one week. The major issue with this drug is that it can actually cause <u>potentially fatal ventricular arrhythmias</u>, especially in patients just starting or re-starting therapy. For this reason, patients receiving this drug must be admitted to a facility for close medical monitoring for a minimum of 3 days when starting or re-starting therapy with this drug.

Clozaril® National Registry

The Clozaril® National Registry is essentially a database where the white blood cell count (WBC) for patients receiving therapy with clozapine can be recorded and viewed. Clozaril® (clozapine) is used in the treatment of various psychiatric disorders (e.g. schizophrenia, bipolar disorder). The problem with clozapine is the <u>potentially fatal side effect of agranulocytosis</u> (suppression of white blood cell production). For this reason, white blood cells must be measured by a medical lab and recorded in the Clozaril® National Registry every week for the first 6 months of therapy and periodically thereafter. Pharmacies can only dispense enough of the drug to treat the patient until their next scheduled lab work (e.g. a 7 days' supply every week for the first 6 months of therapy). This program has been referred to as the "no blood, no drug" program.

Do all REMS programs require as much work as iPLEDGE™, THALIDOMID REMS™, T.I.P.S., and the Clozaril® National Registry?

No, in fact some drugs have REMS programs that are so simple you might be surprised they are considered REMS programs at all. One example is Dulera® (mometasone furoate/formoterol). The only requirement for the Dulera® REMS program is that the increased risk of asthma-related death associated with the use of long-acting beta agonists (such as the formoterol found in Dulera®) must be communicated to healthcare professionals and prescribers.

How does a drug get approved by the FDA for use in humans?
Drugs are approved by the FDA after they are proven to be safe and effective. Proof comes from clinical trial data. Clinical trials are comprised of four phases (see below) and the process of obtaining FDA approval usually takes several years.

Phase 1 Clinical Trials
- Small study involving 20 - 80 healthy male volunteers.
- Low doses are tested.
- Collect data on drug bioavailability and dose needed to elicit a response.

Phase 2 Clinical Trials
- Study involving 40 - 300 patients with the disease of interest.
- Minimum effective dose and maximum toxic dose are determined.
- Record side effects experienced by the test subjects.

Phase 3 Clinical Trials
- Study involving 300 – 3,000 patients of various gender, race, lifestyle, and age.
- Assess the risks and benefits of using the drug.
- Refine the drug formulation.
- Conduct placebo studies.

Post-marketing Surveillance
- Continue to gather information about the safety and effectiveness of a drug after it has been approved and marketed.
- Some drugs get removed from the market due to revelations from post-marketing surveillance (e.g. Vioxx® (rofecoxib) was a COX-2 inhibitor removed from the market when post-marketing surveillance revealed an increased risk of cardiovascular events such as heart attack and stroke).

1) Use tall man lettering

Tall man lettering is a way to emphasize the difference in drug names that otherwise look similar. For instance, Hydroxyzine and Hydralazine are two drug names that, at first glance, look quite similar. When you use tall man lettering, HydOXYzine and HydrALAZINE look less similar, thus reducing the chance that one will be misinterpreted as the other.

Below is a modified list from FDA.gov* which demonstrates the use of tall man lettering in differentiating look-alike/sound-alike medications:

AcetaHEXAMIDE	AcetaZOLAMIDE
BuPROPion	BusPIRone
ChlorproMAZINE	ChlorproPAMIDE
ClomiPHENE	ClomiPRAMINE
CycloSPORINE	CycloSERINE
DAUNOrubicin	DOXOrubicin
DimenhyDRINATE	DiphenhydrAMINE
DOBUTamine	DOPamine
HydrALAZINE	HydrOXYzine
MethylPREDNISolone	MethylTESTOSTERone
NiCARdipine	NIFEdipine
PredniSONE	PrednisoLONE
risperiDONE	rOPINIRole
SulfADIAZINE	SulfiSOXAZOLE
TOLAZamide	TOLBUTamide
VinBLAStine	VinCRIStine

*Source: http://www.fda.gov/Drugs/DrugSafety/MedicationErrors/ucm164587.htm

2) Separate inventory

A popular method for preventing medication dispensing errors is separating inventory. When medications are organized alphabetically, it is common to have drugs with very similar names stored right next to each another on the shelf (e.g. Isosorbide Mononitrate & Isosorbide Dinitrate or Metoprolol Tartrate & Metoprolol Succinate). By separating medications that have similar names, results occur that can contribute to safer dispensing practices. First, since the drugs are stored apart from each other, there is less of a chance that the bottles will get mixed up during storage. Second, the person filling the prescription is forced to stop and think rather than quickly reach for the first drug that appears to be correct. For instance, let's say metoprolol tartrate is stored in alphabetical order with the rest of the drugs, but the metoprolol succinate is stored on another shelf away from the rest of the inventory. When you receive an order to fill a metoprolol prescription, you remember that metoprolol is stored in two different locations. So, before you can fill the prescription, you must figure out which drug to dispense.

3) Use leading zeros

Leading zeros help to ensure accurate translation of numbers less than 1. By omitting a leading zero, you run the risk of causing the patient to receive a dose many times higher than the intended dose. This can be a fatal mistake.

Acceptable: 0.1, 0.005, 0.02, 0.99
Unacceptable: .1, .005, .02, .99

What is the difference between .99 and 0.99?

.99 could easily be misinterpreted as ninety-nine. Consider how detrimental a mistake it could be if a patient was supposed to get 0.99 grams of a drug and they ended up getting 99 grams. One hundred times the prescribed dose could cause serious adverse effects up to and including death.

4) Avoid trailing zeros

While leading zeros can prevent fatal dispensing errors, trailing zeros can cause them. Let's say a patient is prescriber issues a prescription to a patient for: Alprazolam 1 mg PO QID PRN anxiety. When writing the prescription, the prescriber uses a trailing zero, so one milligram is written as "1.0 mg." So the prescription looks like this:

Alprazolam 1.0 mg PO QID PRN anxiety

When reading this prescription, the technician and/or pharmacist might perceive the strength to be ten (10) milligrams instead of one (1) milligram. This misinterpretation could lead to a fatal dispensing error. Never use trailing zeros. Write one as 1, not 1.0 or 1.00.

5) Avoid error-prone abbreviations

Another safety strategy is avoiding the use of error-prone abbreviations. Much like leading and trailing zeros, certain abbreviations can lead to dangerous misinterpretations. The FDA and ISMP* have teamed up in a campaign to eliminate the use of error-prone abbreviations. Below is a list of some common error-prone abbreviations. As a general rule it is best to write out the instructions word for word and avoid abbreviations all together.

Error-Prone Abbreviation	Potential Misinterpretation
AD (right ear)	OD (right eye)
AS (left ear)	OS (left eye)
AU (both ears)	OU (both eyes)
OD (right eye)	AD (right ear)
OS (left eye)	AS (left ear)
OU (both eyes)	AU (both ears)
CC (cubic centimeters)	U (units)
HS (bedtime)	HS (half-strength) or HR (hour)
BT (bedtime)	BID (twice daily)
IU (international units)	IV (intravenous)
IN (intranasal)	IM (intramuscular)
QD or Q1D (daily)	QID (four times daily)
QOD (every other day)	QD (daily) or QID (four times daily)
OD (right eye)	QD (daily)
SC or SQ (subcutaneous)	5 Q ___ (five every)
ss (one-half)	55 (fifty-five)
I/d (one per day)	TID (three times daily)
° (hours; e.g. 6° = 6 hours)	0 (zero; e.g. 60 = sixty)
UD (as directed)	Unit Dose
Per Os (by mouth)	OS (left eye)

*What is the ISMP?

The Institute for Safe Medication Practices (ISMP) is a nonprofit organization that is devoted to preventing medication errors and ensuring safe use of medications.

Each health care organization seeking to satisfy the requirements of the National Patient Safety Goals (a set of requirements that are part of the Joint Commission accreditation* process) has the responsibility to develop a look-alike/sound-alike medication list. Here is an example look-alike/sound-alike list:

Aciphex and Aricept
Advair and Advicor
Alprazolam and Lorazepam
Amlodipine and Amiloride
Benadryl and Benazepril
Bupropion and Buspirone
Celebrex and Celexa**
Celebrex and Cerebyx**
Clomiphene and Clomipramine
Clonidine and Klonopin**
Clozaril and Colazal
Codeine and Lodine
Diprivan and Ditropan
Dobutamine and Dopamine
Durasal and Durezol
Fioricet and Fiorinal
Flonase and Flovent
Fomepizole and Omeprazole
Glyburide and Glipizide
Guaifenesin and Guanfacene
Hydralazine and Hydroxyzine**

Kapidex and Casodex
Keppra and Keflex
Lamictal and Lamisil
Lunesta and Neulasta
Metformin and Metronidazole
Mirapex and Miralax
Misoprostol and Mifespristone
Oracea and Orencia
Oxycodone and Oxycontin
Patanol and Platinol
Pentobarbital and Phenobarbital
Prograf and Prozac
Quinine and Quinidine
Risperidone and Ropinirole
Sitagliptin and Sumatriptan
Tiagabine and Tizanidine
Tramadol and Trazadone**
Vinblastine and Vincristine**
Wellbutrin SR and Wellbutrin XL
Zantac and Zyrtec

*Joint Commission accreditation is intended to be a mark of high quality care. Health care organizations usually seek Joint Commission accreditation because it is a precondition to receiving Medicare and Medicaid payments in many states.
**These are some of the most problematic look-alike/sound-alike names.

High-alert (or high-risk) medications are drugs with a high likelihood of causing serious harm, especially when used improperly. Typically, each institution will compile a list of medications they consider to be in the high-risk category. As a result, the medications that are considered high-risk may vary from one institution to another. Drugs from the following classes usually end up on an institution's high-alert medication list.

Anticoagulants (e.g. heparin, warfarin, enoxaparin)
These drugs are used in the treatment and prevention of blood clots, but they can cause potentially fatal **bleeding** if too much is administered to the patient.

Neuromuscular blockers (e.g. rocuronium, succinylcholine, pancuronium)
These drugs are commonly used to **stop breathing** to allow for mechanical ventilation. These drugs are usually considered to be high-risk since they take away the patient's ability to breathe.

Opioids (e.g. morphine, hydromorphone, fentanyl, meperidine)
These drugs are used to treat pain, but they can cause potentially fatal **respiratory suppression** at high doses.

Insulin (e.g. Humulin®, Novolin®, Humalog®, NovoLog®, Apidra®)
Insulin functions to decrease blood sugar by increasing cellular utilization of glucose in patients with diabetes, but too much insulin can cause a condition known as hypoglycemia*. In severe cases, **hypoglycemia** can be fatal.

*Hypoglycemia means low blood sugar (hypo- = low, -glyc- = sugar, -emia = blood). Symptoms of hypoglycemia include dizziness, confusion, shakiness, sweating, and heart palpitations.

If any of these situations arise, the technician must defer the issue to a pharmacist.

Drug Utilization Review (DUR)
Only a pharmacist can complete a drug utilization review. The purpose of the review is to identify and respond to potential and actual drug interactions, therapeutic duplications, incorrect dosages, drug allergies, apparent drug misuse or abuse, and other medication-related issues that require professional judgment for resolution.

Therapeutic Substitution
Whenever dispensing a medication other than the one the prescriber wrote for (i.e. a generic substitute), a pharmacist must bear the responsibility of making the final decision regarding which formulation will be dispensed.

OTC recommendations
All requests for over-the-counter (OTC) drug recommendations must be deferred to a pharmacist.

Adverse Drug Event (ADE)
A patient/customer complaining of, or asking questions about, an adverse reaction related to use of a medication should have their issue deferred to a pharmacist.

Missed dose
If a patient/customer requests advice from a technician regarding what to do in the case of a missed dose, the technician must defer the request to a pharmacist.

What is the purpose of a material safety data sheet (MSDS)?
Material safety data sheets exist to provide chemical product information.

Specifically, what information does an MSDS provide about a particular chemical product?
- Chemical and physical properties.
- Health, safety, fire, and environmental hazards.
- Information on what to do if the product is accidentally spilled.

The information provided in a material safety data sheet is intended to be used by _____ & _____.
- Workers that will potentially be exposed to the chemicals.
- Emergency response personnel (e.g. firefighters).

Who is responsible for making MSDS's available to you?
Your employer.

True or false. Eye drops can be instilled into the ear to treat conditions of the ear.
True.

True or false. Ear drops can be instilled into the eye to treat conditions of the eye.
False, eye drops are manufactured to be bacteria-free and to contain gentle preservatives. Since the ear is not as sensitive as the eye, ear drops are not as gentle as eye drops. If ear drops are instilled in the eye, the patient will experience burning and irritation of the eye.

Congratulations, you are almost prepared to take the PTCB exam! Before putting an end to your study efforts, I would recommend reviewing the math sections of this book a few more times, especially in the week leading up to the exam. Being successful on the math problems is crucial to passing. When you feel ready to test yourself, consider taking an Official PTCB Practice Exam, available online at <https://app.testrac.com/ptcb/delivery/>.

Tips to help you perform well on the actual exam:
- If you have never been to the testing center before, drive there a day or two prior to the exam so you know exactly how to get there.
- Ensure you are well-rested, well-hydrated, and well-fed on exam day.
- Do not rush through the exam, remain calm.
- The test is multiple-choice, so if you don't know the right answer to a question/problem, then try to eliminate some of the choices you know are wrong.
- When you don't know an answer and you are forced to guess, do not select an answer you have never heard of (e.g. if you have it narrowed down to: "A. Diabetes" or "B. Diffuse Intravascular Coagulation," then choose "A. Diabetes"). The answer is probably easier than you think.

WRITE A REVIEW, HELP A CHILD IN NEED!

Did you have a positive experience using PTCB Exam Simplified? If so, we want to hear about it! When you write a review, we donate $2 to Kids Helping Needy Kids (KHNK), an American-based non-profit organization that provides aid to underprivileged children in Ethiopia. How do you participate? Just complete these two simple steps:

1. Write a review on our Amazon.com product page.
2. E-mail a copy of your review along with the Amazon order number to **customerservice@pharmacylawsimplified.com** with the subject heading "PTCB Exam Simplified Review."

Within a few business days you will receive a donation confirmation e-mail from Kids Helping Needy Kids. It's that easy! Want to learn more about KHNK? Visit **www.khnkp.org!**

Made in the USA
Lexington, KY
24 January 2014